Working with Physicians
in Health Promotion
A Key to Successful Programs

Salvinija G. Kernaghan
Barbara E. Giloth

American Hospital Publishing, Inc.,
a wholly owned subsidiary
of the American Hospital Association

This book was developed under a grant from the Exxon Corporation.

Library of Congress Cataloging in Publication Data

Kernaghan, Salvinija G.
    Working with physicians in health promotion.

    Reprint. Originally published: Chicago, Ill.: American
Hospital Association, c1983.
    Includes bibliographical references.
    1. Health education. 2. Patient education. 3. Physi-
cian and patient. I. Giloth, Barbara E. II. Title.
RA440.5.K47 1984   610'.7   84-2925
ISBN 0-939450-21-6

Catalog no. 070124

Printed in the U.S.A.
1M-9/83-3-1167
1M-5/84-0032
2M-1/85-0072

Audrey Young, Editor, Book Division
Marjorie Weissman, Manager, Book Editorial Department
Dorothy Saxner, Vice-President, Books

CONTENTS

In July 1982, the Exxon Corporation awarded a grant to the Hospital Research and Educational Trust, an American Hospital Association (AHA) affiliate, to fund a pilot project directed by the AHA's Center for Health Promotion. The purpose of this project was to assist health promotion staff to involve physicians more effectively in planning, promoting, and implementing health promotion services. Health promotion practitioners had repeatedly cited "lack of physician support" as a major barrier to successful programming. Yet, while this problem was frequently alluded to in articles and during professional health promotion meetings, no program or publication substantively addressed the various aspects of this complex issue, from its professional and institutional causes to a description of solutions that have worked in a variety of settings. One goal of this project was to develop a resource publication that would accomplish this objective.

During the initial data collection, a major strategy was to identify successful health promotion programs--in particular, the winners of the first National Patient Education Leaders Award program and the participants in the annual conference for Innovators of Community Health Promotion--and to determine how physicians had been involved in various stages of planning and implementing programs at these hospitals. Because of their similarities, not all of these programs are specifically discussed in the text; however, their collective experience provided an important knowledge base for the development of this book. This base was then expanded as an increasing number of health professionals interested in the issue were identified. The strength of the book, we think, lies in its practical and experiential foundation, to which scores of individuals have contributed during the past year.

Although the book was to be, and remains, directed to health promotion staff who wish to involve physicians more effectively in their health promotion programs, our approach to the issue has changed gradually over the course of the year. Our original intention was the identification of various strategies to improve physician involvement in health promotion programs. Our discussions throughout the year with program staff who have successfully worked with physicians, however, suggested that the establishment of a collaborative working relationship with physicians should be the initial basis for various levels of their involvement in program development and implementation. The final title of this book--Working with Physicians in Health Promotion: A Key to Successful Programs--reflects this change.

The preparation of this book reflects the energy of a long list of contributors. Barbara Giloth, patient education manager, Center for Health Promotion, directed the project of which this book is a part. Salvinija G. Kernaghan developed the format for the book, researched the topics to be covered, interviewed numerous physicians and health promotion staff, and wrote the manuscript. Twyjean Owens, project secretary, provided secretarial support to the project and typed the manuscript.

During the early stages of writing this publication a wide variety of individuals were asked to review sample chapters and provide input into the development of the entire manuscript. We would like to thank the following reviewers for their contributions:

Rex D. Archer, M.D., Ann Arbor, MI

Dena Baskin, R.N., coordinator of patient education, Day Kimball Hospital, Putnam, CT

Margaret Bazeley, patient health education coordinator, Veterans Administration Medical Center, Saginaw, MI

Ruth Behrens, senior advisor, Worksite Health Promotion, Office of Disease Prevention and Health Promotion (DHHS), Washington, DC

Sharyn Bills, managing editor, PROmoting HEALTH, Center for Health Promotion, American Hospital Association, Chicago, IL

Deal Chandler Brooks, Division of Medical Affairs, American Hospital Association, Chicago, IL

Christine Brown, R.N., program director, The Well Being, Scripps Memorial Hospital, LaJolla, CA

Jeffrey Burtaine, M.D., wellness project director, Allentown & Sacred Heart Wellness Center, Allenton, PA

William Carlyon, Ph.D., director, Health Education Program, American Medical Association, Chicago, IL

Jean Case, M.D., assistant medical director, Medical and Environmental Health Department, Exxon Corporation, New York, NY

Sandra Cornett, Ph.D., patient education coordinator, Ohio State University Hospitals, Columbus, OH

Katherine Crosson, M.P.H., director, Patient Education Section, The University of Texas Cancer Center, M.D. Anderson Hospital and Tumor Institute, Houston, TX

Elizabeth DuVerlie, director of program development, Maryland Hospital Education Institute, Lutherville, MD

Joseph J. Fanucchi, M.D., director, Occupational Health Service, St. Joseph Hospital, Omaha, NE

Linda Hines, R.N., M.S., clinical specialist, Ambulatory Nursing, University of Maryland Hospital, Baltimore, MD

June Hosick, director, Educational Services, The Christ Hospital, Cincinnati, OH

Janice Hutchinson, M.D., assistant director, Health Education Program, American Medical Association, Chicago, IL

Donald Iverson, Ph.D., director, Health Promotion/Disease Prevention Program, Mercy Medical Center, Denver, CO

Diane Jensen, R.N., assistant director of nursing, Decatur Memorial Hospital, Decatur, IL

Steve Jonas, M.D., M.P.H., associate professor, Department of Community and Preventive Medicine, State University of New York Stony Brook, Stony Brook, NY

Lynn Jones, employee health manager, Center for Health Promotion, American Hospital Association, Chicago, IL

Joann Kairys, health education program coordinator, Hitchcock Clinic, Hanover, NH

Bill Kane, Ph.D., executive vice president, American College of Preventive Medicine, Washington, DC

Mike Kulzycki, director of communications, Hospital Research and Educational Trust, Chicago, IL

Pamela Jean Larson, M.P.H., director of health education, Kaiser Permanente Medical Center-Oakland, Oakland, CA

Josephine Laventhol, director of patient education, Montefiore Hospital & Medical Center, Bronx, NY

Susan Lebergen, community relations representative, Appleton Memorial Hospital, Appleton, WI

Elizabeth Lee, director, Center for Health Promotion, American Hospital Association, Chicago, IL

Mary Longe, community health promotion manager, Center for Health
   Promotion, American Hospital Association, Chicago, IL

Joy Lomax Martin, patient education coordinator, Baptist Memorial
   Hospital, Memphis, TN

Barbara McCool, Ph.D., executive vice president, Strategic Management
   Services, Shawnee Mission, KS

Rose-Marie McCormick, director, Homegoing Education and Literature Program,
   Columbus Children's Hospital, Columbus, OH

Robert McGowan, president, The Institute for Organizational Effectiveness,
   Inc., Manchester, NH

Patricia Mullen, Dr.P.H., associate director, Center for Health Promotion
   Research and Development, Houston, TX

John Mullin, director of exercise physiology, Madison General Hospital,
   Madison, WI

John Nagle, assistant director, Health Promotion/Disease Prevention
   Program, Mercy Medical Center, Denver, CO

Loretta Olsen, R.N., patient teaching coordinator, Bryan Memorial
   Hospital, Lincoln, NE

George Randt, M.D., Center for Health Promotion, Riverside Hospital,
   Toledo, OH

D. Cramer Reed, M.D., senior vice president, Wesley Medical Center,
   Wichita, KS

Jane Root, supervisor, Allied Health, St. Vincent Hospital and Health Care
   Center, Inc., Indianapolis, IN

Denise Shipp, American College of Obstetricians and Gynecologists,
   Washington, DC

Sue A. Stock, Chief of Occupational Therapy, Ingham Medical Center,
   Lansing, MI

Nan Stout, M.P.H., national coordinator for patient education, Veterans
    Administration, Washington, DC

Ann Strong, R.N., patient education coordinator, Norfolk General Hospital,
    Norfolk, VA

Jo Taylor, R.N., patient education coordinator, Piedmont Hospital,
    Atlanta, GA

Malcolm C. Todd, M.D., Long Beach, CA

Carmine Valente, Ph.D., executive director, Center for Health Promotion,
    Inc., Baltimore, MD

Scott Vierke, Ph.D., program manager, Swedish Wellness Systems, Inc.,
    Denver, CO

Ted Warren, Ph.D., director, Division of Education, Stormont-Vail Regional
    Medical Center, Topeka, KS

Suzanne Whitehead, R.N., director, Division of Nursing, American Hospital
    Association, Chicago, IL

Mary Woodrow, director, Health Education Services, El Camino Hospital,
    Mountain View, CA.

In addition to reviewing the manuscript, nine physicians met with project
staff not only to discuss the progress of the book, but to recommend other
activities that could be undertaken by the Center for Health Promotion to
encourage cooperation among hospital health promotion staff and physicians.
We would like to offer special thanks to these advisors for their time and
thoughtful comments.

    Albert M. Antlitz, M.D., Mercy Hospital, Baltimore, MD

    Linda Clever, M.D., director, Department of Occupational Health, Pacific
        Medical Center, San Francisco, CA

    Ronald M. Davis, M.D., immediate past chairperson of the Medical
        Association Medical Student Section, Government Council, Highland, IN

    Merlin K. DuVal, M.D., president and chief executive officer, Associated
        Hospital Systems, Phoenix, AZ

George Jackson, M.D., director, Employee Occupational Health Service, Duke
    University Medical Center, Durham, NC

Mary McLaughlin, M.D., chairperson, Department of Community Medicine, Long
    Island Jewish-Hillside Medical Center, New Hyde Park, NY

David Olive, M.D., immediate past chairperson of the American Medical
    Association Resident Physician Section, Government Council, Durham, NC

John Renner, M.D., director, Sisters of St. Mary Family Medicine Center,
    Kansas City, MO

George T.C. Way, M.D., Poughkeepsie, NY

Many individuals contributed specific examples of their experiences working
with physicians. We would like to thank them collectively here and refer the
reader to Appendix A where their names and addresses are listed to facilitate
follow-up contact.

Finally, we would like to thank several individuals for their unique
contribution to this book and to the entire project. Special thanks to
Ruth Behrens, formerly the director of the AHA's Center for Health Promotion,
who provided the original direction for this project; to Monte DuVal, M.D.,
for his support and encouragement prior to and during its implementation; to
Joseph Fanucchi, M.D., for a manuscript review that directed us most
specifically to the key issues that affect the physician/health promotion
staff relationship; and to Jean Case, Barbara Ciechacki, Loren Kahle, and
Jerrold Weitzman at Exxon for their initial support and useful advice during
the course of the project.

                                        Salvinija G. Kernaghan
                                        Barbara E. Giloth
                                        July 1, 1983

INTRODUCTION

During the past two decades, a variety of social and economic forces have pushed the concepts and practice of health promotion into public view. Many of these same forces have generated increased health promotion activity in hospitals. Not only have traditional patient education efforts been refined and greatly expanded, but hospitals also have moved into new areas of health promotion through community health education and employee health programs.* In all of these efforts, hospitals have found physician support and involvement to be a key factor in a program's utilization and effectiveness.

The continuing influence of physicians on the success of such programs is therefore understandable. Although hospitals have become the primary sponsors of many forms of health promotion, most individuals still look to their primary care-giver, the physician, for advice on how best "to achieve an optimum level of physical and mental health." Their support and involvement is therefore highly desirable. And in some forms of health promotion, such as. in patient education, physician involvement is often crucial, because patients' access to information, training in self-care skills, and ability to change behavior begin with the physician and are integral to effective medical treatment. In turn, how well physicians and other health care professionals teach patients can strongly influence patterns of use of hospital services.

Therefore, it is of some concern to hospitals that many of the health promotion programs they offer lack physician support. When hospital-based educators are asked to describe the problems they most often face in program

---

*According to the definition developed by the American Hospital Association's Center for Health Promotion, "health promotion (including health information and health education) is the process of fostering awareness, influencing attitudes, and identifying alternatives so that individuals can make informed choices and change their behavior in order to achieve an optimum level of physical and mental health and improve their physical and social environment." In particular, patient education is used when the health education is directed to persons, and their families and friends when appropriate, who are either awaiting or undergoing medical treatment. Community health promotion encompasses a variety of health education and health information programs that are offered to individuals who are outside of the health care institutional setting. Employee health programs are designed to help businesses to protect the physical health and safety of employees at the workplace, to assist employees with personal problems that are interfering with job performance, and to encourage employees to change lifestyle habits that may increase their health risks.

implementation, lack of physician support is often reported for all kinds of health promotion programs.* Whatever the motivation physicians may have for withholding their support--from the supposition that no one else is capable of teaching their patients to scepticism about the medical soundness of some health promotion techniques--the challenge that hospitals and their health promotion staffs face is a common one: to involve physicians in health promotion programs, and to do so effectively and appropriately.

The goal of this volume is to help hospital-based educators to work with physicians to meet the challenge. The strategies that the document describes are each meant to encourage a different level of physician support. However, not all of these approaches for generating support are likely to be effective with every physician group, in every institution, or with every health promotion program. An understanding of the factors that influence physicians' responses to specific programs in specific environments must precede any plan to change those responses. Part I of this volume attempts to describe these factors by discussing the attitudes and values that are common to physicians-- regarding the purpose and conduct of medical care, their responsibilities toward their patients, and their responses to the pressures of their own practice. As physicians themselves report in the literature and elsewhere, an understanding of these attitudes can help to alleviate the antagonism that sometimes develops between physicians and those who would impose health promotion programs on them and their clients without previous consultation about interest or need. Such understanding can reveal untapped incentives that could readily engender physician support for health promotion programs; these positive factors are also discussed in Part I of this volume. Finally, the last chapter in Part I describes some of the influences that the environment may impose on physicians that may further color their attitude toward health promotion. These may arise from the immediate environment of the hospital, from physicians' private practices, or from larger state-wide or national sources. An assessment of these factors will help educators to work more effectively with physicians and to develop strategies that may be to their mutual benefit.

The degree to which any of these factors is at work in a specific institution cannot be gleaned from this document. An educator must begin the effort of changing physician attitudes by talking to physicians themselves. The rapport that can be developed by these one-to-one communications will have a direct bearing on the roles that physicians come to play in health promotion

----

*As the AHA definition for health promotion suggests, the term "health promotion program" will be used throughout this book when programs are being discussed generically. Similarly, the term "department" will be used generally to refer to the organizational unit that is responsible for coordinating program development and delivery. Because a wide variety of professionals are responsible for program coordination, we will generally refer to them as "educators." When we discuss particular kinds of programs, we will designate whether they are intended for patient education, community health education, or employee health.

activities. The process of defining the physician's, the educator's, and others' roles in relation to health promotion must clearly be specific to each institution and must depend on consensus-building by the individuals involved, as they exchange and modify their attitudes and concerns. Despite the uniqueness of each institution's physician group and the health promotion needs of its community, guidelines can be offered to help the role definition process. Some of these guidelines have been gathered from the experiences of physicians and educators in a variety of programs that have enjoyed success. Others have been more formally developed by several physicians' groups in an attempt to encourage their members to actively incorporate the concepts of health promotion in their practice. These guidelines and suggestions for defining roles also are discussed in Part I.

How educators can help physicians to act on these role definitions is discussed in Part II. Because each kind of hospital-based, health-related education--whether it be inpatient education, communitywide health promotion in its ever increasing variety, or an employee health program--offers physicians the opportunity to play an assortment of roles, the strategies that are described in Part II are not categorized according to program definitions. Rather, the strategies are discussed according to the level of physician support and involvement they are intended to achieve. This arrangement of the material should help the educator in a given institution to select the approach that is the most promising, no matter what combination of health education elements is planned or what these elements are called.

Finally, the case studies in Part III of this volume describe in more detail several specific methods--the resources they required, the organizational changes that were needed to implement them, and so forth--as these strategies were implemented in particular hospitals. The appendices that follow are designed to guide the educator to further resources: the first lists the names and institutional affiliations of individuals who provided examples and other material for this document; the second describes projects that various organizations are conducting to increase physician involvement in health promotion and to develop tools--protocols, manuals, CME courses, and the like--specifically for physician use; the third is a list of resources published for physicians who wish to incorporate various aspects of health promotion into their practice.

The combination of conceptual material in Part I, the practical strategies in Parts II and III, and the appendices should prove useful to educators who seek physician support in developing sound and effective hospital-based health promotion programs. Although this volume grows out of hospital-based experience and encourages the use of hospital-based networks for involving physicians, the benefits of increased physician support of the concept and practice of health promotion should accrue to the entire community.

PART I

CONCEPTUAL BASIS FOR PHYSICIAN PARTICIPATION
IN HEALTH PROMOTION PROGRAMS

Chapter 1

THE RANGE OF ROLES PHYSICIANS CAN ASSUME IN HEALTH PROMOTION

The relationship between a patient and a physician is the basic unit upon which the health care system is founded. The strength of the relationship depends on several factors, not least of which is the physician's clinical skill in diagnosis and treatment. The degree to which the patient and the physician share the decision-making and the responsibility for the treatment is another important aspect of this relationship. Within this aspect, physicians have a range of options for dealing with the information and health-related counselling needs of patients.

As practitioners in both inpatient and ambulatory care settings, physicians have the opportunity to use the medical encounter "to help patients improve their health status in any way possible."[1] They can be teachers who impart knowledge about an illness and about the tasks patients must perform to treat that illness. In addition, they can play the role of counselor for positive lifestyle change when they discover a connection between the expressed reason for a patient's visit and that patient's health-impairing habits. In the larger institutional setting, physicians' roles as teachers and counselors can be augmented in two major ways. One is through the role of advocate not only of the concepts of health promotion but also of its specific applications through programs the institution sponsors or provides; physicians can help to promote such programs both among their collagues who are not yet convinced of their usefulness and among their patients. Another major role physicians can play in the institution is that of adviser, planner, and participant in the program development process.

The Minimum Level of Involvement

Traditionally, both society and the medical profession have given physicians considerable freedom in either accepting or rejecting these roles--all, that is, but one. Within the physician's broad responsibilities as teacher, society has singled out one responsibility that it has considered important enough to codify in law: the responsibility to inform the patient about the diagnosis and about treatment options and risks and to elicit the patient's consent.

This form of patient education has come to be known as "informed consent." The legal concept of an "informed" patient is a relatively recent one,[2] and the manner in which it is embodied in statutes and their application differs somewhat from state to state. However, as a presidential commission on medical ethics recently concluded, the societal values that underly these legal embodiments are commonly held and of longer standing.[3] "Fundamentally, informed consent is based on respect for the individual, and, in particular, for each individual's capacity and right both to define his or her own goals and to make choices designed to achieve those goals. But in defining informed consent (and its exceptions) the law has tempered this right of self-determination with respect for other values, such as promotion of well-being in the context of an expert-layperson relationship."

Not only society at large but also several of its health care-related
institutions have examined this relationship and have established some
guidelines for the communication that should occur between physician and
patient within the institutional setting. The Joint Commission on the
Accreditation of Hospitals (JCAH), specifically referring to informed consent,
claims for the patient:

> ...the right to reasonably informed decisions involving
> his health care. To the degree possible, this should be
> based on a clear, concise explanation of his condition
> and of all proposed technical procedures, including the
> possibilities of any risks of mortality or serious side
> effects, problems related to recuperation, and
> probability of success. The patient should not be
> subjected to any procedure without his voluntary,
> competent or understanding consent, or that of his
> legally authorized representative. Where medically
> significant alternatives for care or treatment exist,
> that patient shall be so informed.[4]

Although JCAH accords each institution's medical staff and governing body the
right to develop its own policy on informed consent, in accordance with state
requirements, the Commission mandates that evidence of such appropriate
consent be included in a patient's medical records.

The American Hospital Association (AHA) has also included informed consent as
an essential component of its Patient's Bill of Rights.[5] In describing this
document, Ludlam writes, "by setting forth these rights in a single but
complete document, the AHA affirmatively called attention of both the public
and the health care providers to how far and how rapidly the interrelationship
between the patient and the health care provider had changed."[6]

The findings of the President's Commission for the Study of Ethical Problems
in Medicine suggest that the change has been more far reaching in the
conception of the relationship than in its practice. A Louis Harris poll
conducted on the commission's behalf solicited the opinions and experiences of
both patients and physicians with regard to disclosure of information and
sharing of decision making in therapeutic settings. As a summary of the
Harris poll reports, "data show that both physicians and the public agree that
full disclosure concerning diagnosis and treatment is desirable."[7] However,
more physicians reported disclosing information to their patients than
patients reported receiving and discussing that information.

In particular, the commission's observations of activities related to ensuring
informed consent by hospitalized patients demonstrated a great disparity
between concept and practice. Despite the majority of physicians' supporting
the concept of shared decision-making, their practice of informing their
patients in institutional settings "bore little resemblance to the intent of
the legal doctrine. Informed consent was seen as a form to be signed in order
to get permission to proceed, rather than as a process of information exchange
and shared decision-making."

The commission's comprehensive study of the complex issues of informed consent concludes with extensive recommendations for both the legal and medical professions in particular and the health care industry in general. However, many of the recommendations can be implemented only in the long-term. In contrast, a possible short-term solution to the disparity between physicians' attitudes toward and their practice of communicating with their hospitalized patients in particular is only hinted at in the Harris survey results. According to the report, "only 32% [of physicians] agree that the legal requirements for obtaining consent are clear and explicit. Furthermore, three quarters of physicians (76%) frankly admit that they do not know which legal standard for informed consent is applicable in the state in which they practice. In other words, physicians' definition of the role that they can appropriately assume in ensuring informed consent is at best a nebulous one, especially when treatment is to occur in the institutional setting. Under these circumstances, Ludlam writes, "many physicians would prefer to delegate the responsibility for obtaining the informed consent to hospital personnel," although "legally and ethically this is not an answer."[8]

The answer may lie instead in the hospital's providing appropriate support to physicians in assuming their responsibility for informed consent. Such support can emanate from several quarters within the institution. The most logical and primary source may be the medical staff as a body, in its role as arbiter of institutional policy on informed consent. Another logical source may be the hospital's legal staff, which can clarify its state statutes on informed consent and interpret the significance of recent applications.

In either of these circumstances, the education staff of the hospital may be asked or offer to play a supportive role. For example, when the patient health education coordinator at the Veterans Administration Medical Center (Saginaw, MI) asked for medical staff members' opinions in a formal needs assessment survey, "legal issues in patient education" was listed as the most important topic about which physicians wanted information. Organizing a seminar or some other form of information exchange could be an excellent opportunity to support the medical staff in this role and to benefit in turn from the physicians' recognition of that support.

Physicians' acquiring a clearer understanding of the parameters of informed consent could also engender other opportunities for cooperation with educators. Indeed, it may offer some insight to those physicians who think their narrow role in ensuring informed consent is the fullest realization of the patient-physician partnership. Their interest in referring their hospitalized patients to educational programs is likely to increase. And they may find greater need for written materials to support their informing and teaching efforts in office practice. The educator should recognize each of these events as an occasion for demonstrating--but always in the spirit of cooperation--the value of the education department's support in the physician-patient relationship.

Other Appropriate Roles: Beyond Informed Consent

The physician who routinely engages patients in discussing their
health-related patterns of behavior and encourages them to assume health
promoting lifestyles stands at the other end of the continuum of roles
physicians can assume in health promotion. It is very unlikely that
physicians will assume such a role without a personal conviction that health
promoting behavior can indeed make a significant difference to a patient's
well being. Even the physician who believes this can be

> ...in a quandary about how to present and emphasize
> health behaviors in routine medical encounters. The
> challenge of introducing the idea of health promotion
> is enough outside the traditional expectation of
> patients and physicians that all too often it is
> slighted, even avoided. However, part of good clinical
> medicine is sensing the patient's receptivity to
> working on health promotion while pressing for the
> resolution of immediate problems. This type of
> clinical alertness has become important as physicians
> are increasingly attuned to the primary prevention of
> illness.[9]

In recognition of the belief that health promotion is one of the functions of
a primary physician (who, according to Currie and Beasley, is much more than
just a primary care physician), various physicians' organizations have begun
to encourage their members to assume greater roles in teaching and
counselling. The American Academy of Family Practice (AAFP), for example, has
formally recognized that patient education can not only have a salutary effect
on the health of patients but also can help to control costs by preventing
catastrophic episodes of illness and by minimizing the debilitating effects of
chronic disease. Therefore, the AAFP urges that family physicians generally
assume active roles in patient education and that they participate in helping
"to determine the essential elements of patient education that are related to
family practice and the consequent patient education-related roles and tasks
of the physician, ancillary personnel, and the patient."[10]

The American Academy of Pediatrics (AAP) has long urged its members to support
the concepts and practice of preventive medicine and child advocacy. The
Academy has also actively cooperated with government initiatives in child
health and, in 1978, launched a public education campaign that emphasized
accident prevention, nutrition, immunization, and health education.[11]

The American College of Cardiology cooperated with the American Heart
Association, the Centers for Disease Control, and the National Heart, Lung,
and Blood Institute to cosponsor a major conference in the role of the
physician in preventing cardiovascular diseases. The proceedings of the
conference echo the participants' resolution that physicians should play a
more active role in helping to persuade patients and the general public to
reduce cardiovascular risk factors.[12]

The largest American organization of physicians, the American Medical Association (AMA), has made a clear statement about the important relationship between health information and health management: "the provision of patient education services designed to assist the patient and his family in the effective management of individual health is a shared and continuous responsibility of both the physician and the patient." The AMA definition of the functions of a primary care physician includes that of personal and family counselling. Finally, since a 1980 resolution was passed by the AMA House of Delegates, the organization has taken on the responsibility to support physicians' activities in health-related education for kindergarten through age 12.[13]

The range of roles that these organizations advocate for physicians in health promotion activities can all be appropriately implemented in a particular institution, given a reasonably responsive corps of physicians and a resourceful education staff. Even in the best of situations, finding such a group is not necessarily easy. For example, among the 44 institutions that were most recently judged to be innovators in the field of health promotion, approximately half reported lack of enthusiasm for health promotion among their medical staffs.[14] Nonetheless, 23 of these programs were able to identify at least one physician who has entered into a more formal relationship with the department or program, in a position that is variously identified as medical advisor, medical education director, or chairman of the health education committee. As this latter title suggests, more than one physician can be drawn into a formal relationship with a program; besides the chairman, other physicians can serve as members of an organized advisory committee for planning and developing programs. As they become more involved in and familiar with the practice of health promotion, these physicians will be able to help the education staff to better define the roles that other physicians in that hospital may be willing to play.

As the opening of this chapter indicates, these roles will tend to fall into three general categories--planning and advising, promoting programs, and actual teaching. For the purpose of a hospital-based health promotion program, physicians' input into program planning and development may be the most essential. Whether the educational strategy is one-to-one instruction, group teaching, written material for self-instruction, audiovisual, or a combination of these, physicians are unlikely to recommend its use to patients unless they find the contents to be accurate, the approach consistent with their own, and the delivery respectful of their relationship with their patients. These elements are best assured if physicians join the program development process. The health promotion staff can create opportunities for physician input--such as eliciting information about physicians' own needs for various teaching materials and about their patients' needs, encouraging physicians to join in planning of programs, and asking them to review materials; how such opportunities can be provided is described in greater detail in Chapter 5 and 6, in Case 2 on conducting surveys, and in Case 3 on working with committees.

Physicians, once convinced that their patients can benefit from appropriate health promotion offerings, will very likely want to refer them to such programs. To facilitate their doing so, the education staff can choose from another set of strategies--such as providing accurate schedules and descriptions of program elements, establishing in-house referral techniques, and helping train physicians' office staff members to inform patients about appropriate programs. Examples of such strategies are described in Chapter 7.

Finally, the health promotion staff in a hospital can be of great help to a physician who wishes to assume more of a teaching role with patients both in the hospital and in the office. Helping to identify sources of teaching materials, organizing workshops for developing effective teaching skills, offering training sessions to prepare physicians' office staff to better support physicians' teaching efforts--these are a few of the strategies that may be appropriate in encouraging physicians in a given community to expand their teaching roles; these examples and others are described further in Chapter 8.

Not all of these suggestions will be appropriate for every institution. Neither will all--or even some--of them be effective in engaging every member of the medical staff. The educators in a given hospital will need to collaborate with their physician-advocates to choose and apply those strategies that appear to be most pertinent and most promising, given the needs of the community, the characteristics of the medical staff, and the resources of the hospital. Setting unrealistic goals for engaging every physician as advocate and promoter and teacher will likely do more harm than good in the effort to build alliances with the medical staff. Not all physicians will want to play all these roles. However, whether they do it well or not, most physicians will insist on retaining their traditional ideal role as primary teacher to the patient. As one physician puts it, "for health educators to position themselves as the teachers and the physicians as the technicians is to pose an insoluble conflict."[15] If instead, he continues, educators posed themselves as coordinators of and "additional teachers to the teaching function and if they tried to stroke the teaching-ness out of every physician," their health promotion programs--and patients--would fare much better.

References

1. Currie, B., and Beasley, J. Health promotion in the medical encounter, in Health Promotion: Principles and Clinical Applications. R. Taylor, ed. Norwalk, CT: Appleton-Century-Crofts, 1982.

2. Ludlam, J. Informed Consent. Chicago: American Hospital Association, 1978.

3. President's Commission for the Study of Ethical Problems in Medicine and Biomedical and Behavioral Research. Making Health Care Decisions. Volume One: Report. Washington, DC: The Commission, 1982.

4. Joint Commision on the Accreditation of Hospitals. Accreditation Manual for Hospitals. Chicago: JCAH, 1982.

5. American Hospital Association. A Patient's Bill of Rights. Chicago: the AHA, 1972.

6. Informed Consent.

7. Making Health Care Decisions.

8. Informed Consent.

9. Health Promotion.

10. National Task Force on Training Family Physicians in Patient Education. Patient Education: A Handbook for Teachers. Kansas City, MO: The Society of Teachers of Family Medicine, 1979.

11. American Hospital Association, Center for Health Promotion and U.S. Dept. of Health and Human Services: Statements About the Health Education Roles and Responsibilities of Selected Health Care Providers. Atlanta, GA: The Association and DHHS, 1981.

12. Proceedings of the 11th conference: prevention of coronary heart disease (September 27-28, 1980, Bethesda, MD). American Journal of Cardiology. 47:713-776, March 1981.

13. Carlyon, P. Physician's Guide to the School Health Curriculum Process. Chicago, IL: American Medical Association, Revised edition, 1983.

14. Unpublished data from applications to Fifth Annual Conference for Innovators of Community Health Promotion, sponsored by the Center for Health Promotion, American Hospital Association, 1983.

15. Batalden, P., M.D. Personal communication, June 2, 1983.

Chapter 2

PHYSICIANS' CURRENT INVOLVEMENT IN HEALTH PROMOTION: DEFINING AND UNDERSTANDING THE PROBLEM

This entire book is based on the premise that the most effective health promotion programs, those that have a positive, long-term impact on patients' health, can boast of active physician support. As the previous chapter suggests, physicians can extend such support by assuming several roles: by doing the teaching themselves and by having and helping others do it. When their physicians choose not to play these roles, some individuals can be put to a great disadvantage. In general, most individuals find their options for participating in their own care and for enhancing their own health at least limited if their physicians neglect the health promotion aspects of their care. Hospitals that offer health promotion programs discover that physician disinterest may mean, at best, a disatisfyingly low rate of use; at worst, it may result in wasted effort and program failure.

Current Level of Physician Involvement

Despite consumers' and hospitals' need for medical input, considerable evidence suggests that they both get less support than they would like in their efforts toward health promotion. The American College of Chest Physicians (ACCP) found, for example, that 80 percent of physicians responding to a College survey had not made a practice of advising their patients to stop smoking.[1] Another survey commissioned by the American Cancer Society (ACS) disclosed that, among 804 persons interviewed (almost half of whom had had a medical checkup during the previous year), only 12.5 percent could recall discussing early signs of colorectal cancer with a physician during that time.[2] According to a spokeman of ACS, early detection of this disease, like that of many others, and the success of subsequent treatment depend not only on patients' awareness of early warning signs but also "on doctors' awareness of their influence on patients' behavior." For example, 70 percent of smokers who responded to the ACCP survey on smoking said that they would attempt to stop smoking if their physicians advised them to do so.

Of equal concern are statistics that suggest major lapses in physician-patient communications even within the context of discussions about specific diagnosis, prognosis, and treatment. According to the President's Commission for the Study of Ethical Problems in Medicine, "the proportion of physicians who report disclosing case and treatment information to their patients is greater than the proportion of the public who report that their physicians discuss these matters with them. In most instances, there is a large and consistent difference of approximately 15-25 percentage points" between the two groups' reporting on such specific matters as diagnosis and prognosis (physicians say they discuss this 90% of the time, while patients say it occurs only 78% of the time); on the nature and purpose of treatment (physicians, 98%; patients, 78%); and on the pros and cons of recommended treatment (physicians, 84%; patients, 68%).[3]

In comparison to such data that describe physicians' doing the teaching themselves, information about their supporting others' work in health promotion is only anecdotal. Nevertheless, the accumulation of anecdotes, especially about hospital-based health promotion activities, is weighty enough for drawing some conclusions: there are many programs that are successful enough, but that could offer benefits to more individuals, if physicians would only refer them. Other programs are languishing for want of physician input into program content or physician approval of a finished product. Finally, some health promotion efforts, especially in such relatively new areas as wellness and occupational health, are often confronted with active opposition from some or most of the medical practitioners who serve a given community.

The educator who must deal with this kind of a response—or lack of response, as the case may be—has two choices. One is to ignore it and try to operate a program without physician support; for many programs, this route is likely to lead nowhere. It is also an ill-fated precedent to set, because it may engender even more negative feelings among the physician group and make the task of launching a future program that much more difficult. The other alternative—and probably the only viable one—is to try first to identify exactly which programs or aspects of programs physicians do not support and then to discover why.

Understanding the reasons for an individual physician's or a medical staff's opposition to a program is crucial for two important reasons. First, their opinion may be based on an accurate judgement that some aspect of the program needs revision. If their judgement is based on a misconception, then it must be corrected. Second, understanding physicians' attitudes toward a particular health promotion program is the basis for developing a dialogue with them about its use by their patients.

Attitudes That Pose Barriers

A recent and telling bit of research about physicians' attitudes toward health promotion describes how one group of physicians report personally adopting health promoting habits. Glanz and her co-authors [4] asked 296 physicians to assess their own health-related behavior according to the seven health practices that were identified in the well-known Alameda County Study: (1) exercising, (2) not smoking, (3) limiting alcohol consumption, (4) sleeping an average of 7-8 hours every night, (5) controlling one's weight, (6) eating breakfast, and (7) seldom eating snacks. The researchers then attempted to relate this set of behaviors, as well as the added practice of an annual medical check-up, to a set of attitudes or beliefs about health. One finding established an obvious relationship between belief and practice: those physicians who believed that a healthy lifestyle has a positive influence on one's health tended to behave accordingly. The more interesting finding, however, suggested that physicians who had experienced illness themselves were those more likely to adopt health-maintaining behaviors. As the authors suggest, "it appears that predispositions to adopt good health habits may be affected more by having personally experienced health problems than by medical knowledge of their efficacy."

Just as personal experiences influence physicians' own health-related habits, so do they also influence physicians' commitment to teaching their patients the basics of self-care and health promotion. There is evidence, for example, that physicians' counselling habits are associated with their own personal health practices; that is, those physicians who smoke are less likely to counsel their smoking patients on this topic, reports Charles Lewis, M.D., professor of medicine, University of California, Los Angeles, School of Medicine.[5] Beyond these, one must consider the experiences that are common to most physicians. They begin with medical school, where students are "engrossed in the intellectual exercises [that are] concerned with pathology" and where most of them are "educated in and oriented to a system that exposes them to patients who for the most part are seriously ill."[6] In the majority of these situations, the young physician's objective is to alleviate a crisis, to apply an immediate solution--to do something to the patient. Therefore, the interventions the physician learns to use are usually those that are proven to benefit the patient and to do so as soon as possible.

Few health promotion interventions can achieve these objectives. Having learned to demand rigorous evidence of the medical interventions they apply, physicians expect the same kind of proof of effectiveness from health promotion measures. Some health promotion measures have simply not been tested enough, for long enough. Others can offer evidence, but it may not be so rigorous as physicians wish. Often, the evidence that is there and is sound does not appear in the literature that physicians tend to read. Educators may also overlook its availability, and so they may not be prepared to support the programs they propose with the kind of evidence that physicians demand. Physicians may also consider health promotion interventions ineffectual for several other reasons. The question of what works in medicine is often related to how much of the intervention must be applied to gain the desired, predictable effect. Much more evaluation research on health promotion intervention will need to be conducted before standardization can be expected both in the intervention and in the dose that must be applied to treat a person's particular need for counselling, for acquiring a self-care skill, and so forth. Even after the intervention is applied, the patient has the option to nullify it--by not following instructions, by not changing habits, etc.; the patient does not have this option with many medical interventions (such as an injection or surgery), and so the probability is much greater that a medical intervention proven effective in clinical trials will alleviate a problem in practice.

The urgency that passing time imposes on a patient-physician encounter is also an important issue, for the physician as well as the patient. Once medical school is completed and a physician begins private practice, determinations of which interventions to apply are made not only on the basis of the life-threatening character of the patient's major problem; they are also made on the basis of the sheer volume of patients waiting to be seen before the end of each day's office hours. "It is a simple equation--the number of minutes available for care divided by the number of patients equals amount of time per patient."[7]

The physician who does take the time to question and counsel the patient regarding health-related habits expects to see some benefits resulting from that investment. Such positive results often do not become apparent--for at least two reasons. One may be that either the physician or the patient or both do not give a new behavior enough time to be established and to make a difference. Another reason physicians often do not see the benefits of health promotion is that they are not really doing health promotion. Many physicians did not learn its principles in medical school and have seldom had the opportunity to acquire them elsewhere. Therefore, they believe that a brief discussion with a patient about some health-impairing habit and one recommendation that the patient try to substitute some more positive behavior constitutes an effective, health promoting intervention.

In this way, the nihilistic stance that health promotion bears little fruit tends to be reinforced. In some physicians, this stance appears in a somewhat modified form: these physicians believe that health promotion--especially the kind that depends on the patient assuming more responsibility (e.g., stopping smoking, wearing seat belts, and such others)--is not a medical problem. Indeed, many of them believe that dealing with these issues is a social responsibility to be addressed by institutions other than medicine. This attitude is clearly related to the traditional medical role of taking responsibility for those interventions that one understands and can control; it permits the patient more to comply with instruction than to participate and share responsibility.

Many of the attitudes that inhibit physicians' advocating health promotion behaviors to their patients also incline these physicians to oppose other health professionals' offering health promotion programs to their patients. The issue of time continues to be an important one, but in a different way; it most often appears as expressed lack of time to join with other health professionals in planning and developing programs. In some cases, however, physicians may use this reason to mask other--probably stronger--barriers to their supporting these programs.

At least two of these barriers arise from physicians' desire to control all aspects of patient care that have traditionally been considered within "the practice of medicine." The first is reluctance to delegate part of a patient's care to another person or to share it. This feeling of duty may seem excessive in some physicians and so narrow as to exclude others from contributing to a patient's well being. Nevertheless, it is based on a sound principle of medical training that attempts to instill in every physician acceptance of responsibility for directing a patient's care. It is inconceivable to most physicians that a health care system could provide effective service without ultimate responsibility for medical care residing in professionals with medical training.

Physicians do accept--indeed, they claim--ultimate responsibility. Very few of them claim all responsibility, however, and so, to one degree or another they accept the contributions that nurses, pharmacists, and various therapists make to a patient's care. Unlike the educator in the hospital, however, these health professionals have a comparatively long history of hospital practice; furthermore, what these professionals do is quite visible and understandable. Most educators cannot claim a similar record--sometimes not for themselves as professionals, sometimes not for the programs that they would like to implement. In many institutions, they may be the newest members of the hospital team; until physicians recognize educators' right to be there, the services they have to offer will also be suspect.

They will be especially suspect if physicians view them as competitive with their own private practice: this is the second barrier that is related to the issue of control. As one physician summarizes the problem in relation to community and occupational health programs, "I doubt there is a significant difference [among physicians] in the general unwillingness...to accept as 'good for my patients' a program which by the admission of most of its supporters is (1) attempting to provide a service which has traditionally--for better or worse, and however much it may not be provided at all--been under the control of physicians; and (2) attempting to better the financial and public-relations position of the institution providing it. In other words, if the reason the program exists is to bring patients (and therefore money) and community goodwill (and therefore money) to the hospital, that may be a legitimate reason for the hospital to develop and promote the program. It's a legitimate business venture. But as a business venture, it does compete with physicians for an ultimately limited number of health care dollars."[8]

Environmental Disincentives to Physicians' Support

Concern about health care dollars also comes into play when a physician considers implementing various kinds of health promotion programs in private practice. Current third party reimbursement patterns do not encourage the physician to do much more than diagnose and treat a patient, and then get on to the next one. A recent study of the attitudes and health promotion practices of 490 Massachusetts-based primary care practitioners reports that financial reimbursement would be the second most valuable type of assistance they would want for increasing their health promotion efforts.[9] Until that happens, a physician who is interested in providing more than minimal information to patients must often cover the cost of the service by stretching the same patient care dollar that has not included the expense until now. That expense may take the form of additional office staff time to provide patient education or to counsel patients in health maintaining measures. Or, at the least, the expense may represent the purchase of educational materials to be distributed to patients in the office.

Even this latter strategy for teaching patients may be a considerable barrier to some physicians--both in terms of time and money. Appropriate materials-- matched to a patient population according to content--are not easy to locate, especially for one who is unfamiliar with educational materials catalogues and with the mysteries of assessing readability. Again, it is not within physicians' normal training or experience to do these tasks, and so they are difficult to incorporate into physicians' daily long-standing habits of providing patient care. Most educators know that considerable health promotion literature is available and how to find it. Most physicians do not. And so it is that "lack of appropriate literature" is one of their most frequently reported reasons for not doing more health promotion. In the Massachusetts study,[10] for example, one-quarter of the physicians cited availability of literature as the kind of assistance that they would find most valuable.

When the health promotion program is delivered by someone other than a physician, someone who is a hospital employee, another set of environmental factors tends to discourage physician support. One of these may be the kind

of relationship--cooperative vs. antagonistic, and all the shades between--
that a physician has with the institution. Another may be a conservative
medical staff organization that exerts a strong pressure on its members to
conform to traditional roles themselves and to demand the same of other health
care professionals who work with them. This latter influence can be
especially strong in patient education programs in which nurses are meant to
be the primary teachers but often find their efforts nullified both by
physicians and by some of their own nursing colleagues. These and other
organizational factors will be discussed further in Chapter 4.

Suffice it to say here that physicians do not create barriers to effective
health promotion by themselves. Not only does their training and experience
often mold them for a role that in effect excludes health promotion. They are
also too often needled and pushed into that role by other health professionals
as these attempt to carve out larger patient care roles for themselves. The
physician who is used to being "captain of the ship" may find the transition
to being a member of "the health care team" very difficult to make, especially
when he is unfamiliar with how well the other team members have been trained.

The patient too may find the concept of "health care team" disorienting;
unfortunately, in some cases, the patient's perception that care becomes more
fragmented than comprehensive is quite correct. In such instances, he may
look to the attending physician to shield him from the barrage of too many
intruders, especially if some of them suggest that the patient too become part
of the team. Many individuals are as set in the traditional physician-patient
relationship as some physicians are, and will prefer to deal only with their
physicians and their directives.

Therefore, educators who wish to change physicians' habits and attitudes
toward health promotion must recognize that they themselves may become one of
the barriers to physician support--even as they attempt to scale the other
barriers that may be more obvious. In the end, the stance of the educator may
be the key to successfully involving physicians in health promotion. If an
educator's first approach says, "cooperate with me, or I'll do it without
you," a great deal of ground is already lost. The hospital cannot afford to
take such a position vis-a-vis its medical staff--both for the sake of its
mission and for the sake of its economic security. Neither can the
hospital-based educator. Generating physician support must be viewed as a
long-term process, not as a series of win-lose events when each new program is
"ready" to be launched. A spirit of cooperation and consensus-seeking is
therefore more promising in removing barriers that have traditionally kept
physicians from supporting health promotion programs. Equally as useful may
be a determination to see the process through, even after a few rejections--
the willingness to continue asking questions, to keep looking for points of
agreement, and so to make certain the door stays open until the next time.

References

1. News item. Capsules, the Newsletter of the Louisiana State Medical
    Society. January 1983, p.5.

2. Patients talk about colorectal cancer-but often not with their doctors.
    Medical World News. Dec. 6, 1982, p. 35.

3. President's Commission for the Study of Ethical Problems in Medicine and Biomedical and Behavioral Research. <u>Making Health Care Decisions.</u> <u>Volume One: Report</u>. Washington, D.C.: The Commission, 1982.

4. Glanz, K., and others. Physicians' health beliefs, health practices, and health status: a survey. A paper presented to the Association for Social Sciences in Health at the Annual Meeting of the American Public Health Association; Montreal, Canada, Nov. 17, 1982.

5. Lewis, C. Personal communication. June 6, 1983.

6. Pratt, H. S. The physician as health educator. <u>Hospital Medical Staff.</u> 4:1-7, Dec. 1975.

7. The physician as health educator.

8. Fannucchi, J. Personal communication. March 1, 1983.

9. Wechsler, H., and others. The physician's role in health promotion--a survey of primary care practitioners. <u>The New England Journal of Medicine.</u> 308:97-100, Jan. 13, 1983.

10. The physician's role in health promotion.

Chapter 3

INCENTIVES FOR PHYSICIAN INVOLVEMENT IN HEALTH PROMOTION

For almost every reason that discourages physicians from supporting health promotion, there is a counter-balancing incentive for them to embrace its concepts both in their own practice and in the work of other health professionals. Of course, these incentives tend to effect more active support if they are operating in a climate that has already shown flexibility in response to change. In turn, this responsiveness depends on a sense of cooperation and trust that has been generated among the major players in an organization—whether these be the physicians, nurses, and office staff in a private practice or the medical staff, the board of trustees, the administration, and the other professionals in a health care institution. Much can be said about the influence of the environment of practice on the way an individual physician or a medical staff will tend to respond to a proposed change—such as a new cardiac rehabilitation program or a wellness center to be affiliated with a hospital. More will be said about this important set of influences in the following chapter. Whatever the configuration of these influences may be, however, the potential incentives for physicians' involvement in health promotion programs will be the same. And they will tend to spring from three basic tenets of the medical profession in general—the physician's commitment to a scientific basis for patient care, the physician's interest in providing high quality care, and the physician's resolve to establish a successful practice.

Commitment to a Scientific Basis for Care

Of all the motives for physicians' rejecting health promotion programs, the one that is least open to question, and the one that they express most frequently and firmly is the lack of evidence that a particular program has a strong enough scientific basis and is therefore likely to deliver the benefits it promises. A complicating factor for a health promotion program is that it must offer two types of evidence: 1) epidemiologic research that links a behavior such as smoking with disease, or a behavior such as exercise with improved health; and 2) behavioral or educational research that suggests that a "stop smoking" program will actually help individuals to stop smoking.

While documentation of the epidemiologic base for lifestyle change has increased, and there is now more evidence of the effectiveness of different types of programs ("stop smoking," for example), it is in the patient education arena that the positive evidence from educational research is most comprehensive. For example, a recent quantitative review of 34 controlled studies demonstrated that, on the average, surgical or coronary patients who were provided information or emotional support to help them deal with a medical crisis did better than patients who received only ordinary care.[1] The same report also reviewed 13 studies that used hospital days post-surgery or post-heart attack as outcome indicators; on the average, such intervention reduced hospitalization by approximately two days below the control group's average of 9.92 days. Results from a five-year followup of hypertensive patients in eight experimental and control groups documented that the hypertensive-related mortality rate was 53.2 percent less for the experimental groups who experienced one or more health education interventions.[2]

Most research related to health promotion programs and outcomes is not reported in the publications most widely read by physicians. Also, because of the nature of educational interventions (that is, not quantifiable, as are units of medication), the new research cannot often provide definitive answers but rather suggest patterns of action that may be productive. However, educators need not rely on others' research to establish the efficacy of health promotion. To show physicians that a new practice will actually benefit patients, health promotion staff should include some evaluation of results in every program design: not only would this tend to assure the quality of a program, it could also raise the level of physician referrals. In many cases, physicians observe that their patients who participate in education programs do better. At least some physicians will always be impressed by data that show their patients or the hospital's patients who participate in educational programs are stopping smoking, are less anxious, are keeping their follow-up appointments, and so forth. Such data may impel physicians not only to intensify their own efforts in advising and teaching patients; such program results should also impel more physicians to subscribe to the concepts of health promotion and to come to rely on other professionals' skills in effecting behavior change.

For some physicians, evidence of a program's effectiveness is a moot point if that program is designed for the well rather than the sick--in other words, if it fits more in the category of a "wellness" program than of patient education. Despite their commitment to scientifically sound courses of treatment, many physicians' view of their own role will continue to be strongly influenced by the medical model. Some physicians will therefore tend to limit their interventions--and those of other health care professionals--to care of acute and chronic illness and so to exclude preventive measures. For these physicians, other incentives may be more relevant--especially if the appeals are made by their patients or by their colleagues.

Interest in High Quality Care

As some of the strategies described in Part II will suggest, physicians may sometimes be better convinced to change their own practices if their patients--rather than some hospital employees--are doing the convincing. Patients who ask questions, and continue to ask them until they get an answer, can be effective change agents for health promotion. As more of the population gets more information about health from the major media, more questions are coming to mind; many of these questions are being asked of the physician, still the most trusted source of medical information. "Informed" patients can be--as often as not--a thorn in the side of the busy physician, because some of them come armed with misinformation from the latest newspaper article or with extravagant expectations generated by the morning "talk" show. Although such patients may constitute an incentive only by coincidence, their need for correct and realistic information is an appeal that no physician can or should deny. If a medical practice begins to see more and more of such patients, its physicians may feel impelled to provide the information these patients seek in a more organized way.

Several examples described in Part II may suggest to educators how they can help physicians be more responsive to these queries and therefore ensure that their patients are operating on information that will help rather than harm them. In these instances, all three parties reap mutual benefit: the patient gets the right information, the physician wins the patient's confidence, and the educator becomes a valuable resource to both, probably to be consulted again.

It is also highly probable that more physicians would practice health promotion if they had the skills. For example, the 490 primary-care physicians who responded to a survey on their health promotion beliefs and practices "expressed little confidence in their current success in helping patients change their behavior. Only 3 to 8 percent thought that they were 'very successful' in helping patients acheive changes in behavior."[3] However, if these physicians were given appropriate support, "...a considerably higher proportion were optimistic about their ability to help patients exercise (21 percent), diet (20 percent), stop smoking (14 percent), manage stress (14 percent), and modify drug use (12 percent) and drinking habits (11 percent)." The types of support they valued most included training in specific subjects (such as alcohol, exercise, and nutrition—23 percent) and in behavior modification (17 percent). Most valuable (40 percent) was information on where to refer patients. These results strongly suggest that not only evidence of a program's effectiveness but also having the opportunity to learn the skills of program delivery may be welcome assistance for some physicians.

The influence of physicians themselves on one another's practice can also be a strong motivator. Their informal exchange of information, anecdotes, and news about innovative methods has always been an important form of continuing education. Any given network of physicians tends to have its favorite few who are consistently dependable sources of information about changes in the state of the art, among other issues. The more often a new technique is described in a positive light by one physician to another, the more quickly that technique will tend to be incorporated into the latter physician's practice. The desire to provide care that meets current standards of medical practice can be a strong incentive for many physicians, especially because the achievement of that desire benefits both the patient and the care-giver.

If desire is not a strong enough motive, some more formal mechanisms are available to encourage physicians to consistently incorporate at least one kind of health promotion into their patient management techniques. A variety of patient education strategies—for example, teaching diabetic patients the techniques of appropriate self-care—have generally been accepted as valuable additions to the management of particular patient populations. These strategies often increase the potential of a given treatment regimen for ensuring a patient's timely recovery. As such, they are important components to include in developing a protocol for treatment and for retrospective audit of that treatment. As physicians have used the quality assurance mechanism to evaluate the quality of other components of patient care, so also have they begun to consider the contribution that patient education can make to assuring that quality. And though the trend is yet to be documented, there is evidence to suggest that patient education is beginning to be discussed more often at QA committee deliberations; some examples of patient education departments' input into these discussions appear in Part II and in Case 1 on quality assurance.

The notion of assuring quality also is clearly related to the concept of reducing risk--especially the risk that some aspect of patient care may harm a patient if it is delivered incorrectly or if it is neglected. An important objective of the function of risk management, certainly an objective to which most physicians can subscribe, is the reduction of costs that are associated with malpractice insurance and litigation. Although the process of ensuring a patient's informed consent is an essential component in risk management, it is not the only one. Neither is it enough to provide patient care that meets the current technical standards. Patients and their families, the final judges of the quality of care that they perceive has been provided, do not feel that the healing process has been completed "until their anxieties, as well as their symptoms, are gone....The patient's perception of medical outcome as claimable incident [in a malpractice suit] is always filtered through attitudes and beliefs...about medicine, regardless of whether these are misconceptions. Whether these assumptions are correct or not, they nonetheless contribute to the patient's personal explanation of what's wrong with him, and to his expectations of what appropriate treatment should be."[4] Physicians who understand this will feel an added economic incentive to communicate more effectively with patients and to engage other relevant professionals to do so. The physicians who are not aware of the relationship between teaching patients and risk reduction may be brought to the realization by the risk management activities of the institution in which they practice. (See Case 1 for examples.)

Another form of incentive that is similar to quality assurance and has recently been introduced also promises to foster the use of patient education as an important component of patient care. Variously called "economic grand rounds," "cost-awareness rounds," or "clinico-economic or cost-awareness conference," this mechanism is designed to address not only the quality of patient care but also its economic consequences. Of course, much research would need to be done before even some of the established forms of patient education are shown to be cost-effective. However, there is enough evidence to suggest that some of these do reduce the costs of hospitalization. For example, as the previously described review by Mumford and others reports, preoperative teaching has been shown to reduce post-operative inpatient days.[5] In the sense that a patient's rapid recovery requires shorter hospitalization, less medication, and generally fewer other health care resources, the issues of quality of care and cost-effectiveness are closely intertwined.

Resolve to Establish a Successful Practice

To consider that such mechanisms as quality assurance, risk management, and economic grand rounds can be effective incentives for physician involvement is to assume that physicians need to cooperate with their community's health care institutions as much as those institutions need to cooperate with physicians. A number of factors may tend to intensify or moderate this need, and these will be discussed further in Chapter 4. Suffice it to say here that the current economic climate is forcing those who pay for health care services to more than ever impose cost control measures on the health care system. Although most of these measures are designed to directly affect hospitals, hospitals are in turn developing ways to share the economic burden of cost control with their medical staffs.

For example, with the advent of such reimbursement methods as cost-per-case and DRG (disease-related group), hospitals may seek ways to work with physicians to develop treatment regimens that fall within imposed cost limits. In such situations, patient education that can reduce inpatient days promises to become an essential component of practice. In like manner, hospitals that are being pressured by local industry, especially through their strong health care coalitions, to provide expanded preventive and primary care will also be impelled to seek relationships with physicians who demonstrate a health promotion philosophy. Some of these coalitions are "evaluating and selecting health education programs to help employees be better medical consumers and looking at education programs in special areas such as stress management and cardiovascular risk."[6] Although some physicians may feel that such developments are more like negative pressure than positive incentive, it is very likely that the economic viability of some physicians' private practices will depend even more on the extent and quality of their relationships with the health care institutions in their communities.

The success of their practices will also continue to depend on physicians' ability to attract and keep patients. To the extent that some patients will still have a free choice of physicians, they will be interested in establishing relationships with those physicians who distinguish themselves in some positive way from others who are practicing in a community. Health promotion programs that physicians offer in their offices or through the hospital where they practice may become a strong marketing tool. Many of these programs are of special interest to middle- and upper-income groups, whose communities often have more physicians per capita than average and where competition among those physicians is thereby intensified.

The ability to expand one's practice base is often diminished if a physician's practice is already saturated with established patients who need only routine, follow-up management. Patient education provided by non-physician staff can permit the physician to use time more efficiently, to assure that patients are getting the education they need, and to open the physician's schedule for more new patients. For example, a study of diabetic care at the Hitchcock Clinic, a group practice in Hanover, NH, disclosed that 90 percent of total diabetes care time was devoted to follow-up care; that 5 percent of the physicians' care time was used for non-compensated patient teaching by telephone; that patients waited two to six weeks for routine care appointments; and new patients waited as long as 10 weeks for initial visits.[7] The recommendations of this study should suggest to other physicians some changes they might consider in their own practice--that is, the addition of a diabetes nurse coordinator, who was to be responsible for routine follow-up care and patient education. "The expected results of this new program included major increases in the productivity of the endocrine section (such as a doubling of new diabetic patients seen by physicians per week) and decreases in patients waiting time for new and return appointments. The detailed cost analysis for this program suggested that the additional salary costs for the nurse coordinator would be more than offset by increased patient visit revenue."

Having found that an illness-preventing, health promotion approach attracts patients, physicians may also find that it helps to keep them as long-term clients. A variety of studies have been conducted to examine the relationship between doctor-patient communication patterns and patient satisfaction. For example, one study was designed to assess the impact of prescriptions on doctor-patient interaction. In contrast to the long-standing myth that most patients "just want the doctor to give me a pill," patients interviewed in this study reported more satisfaction with the communicative aspects of their visits to physicians when they did not receive a prescription.[7] The research concluded that "prescriptions may hinder patient satisfaction with the doctor-patient interaction by substituting for other, more 'meaningful' communication between patient and provider." Another study also reports that the effectiveness of patient/physician communication is related to physicians' tendencies to prescribe medication. "Patients whose physicians correctly estimated their discomfort or pain were more likely to receive prescriptions than patients whose physicians underestimated their discomfort or pain."[8] The latter group, the study reports, "were most likely to report dissatisfaction with the treatment given." Although the findings of these two studies may at first seem contradictory, the variable in both that is directly related to patient satisfaction is not the physician's tendency to write a prescription but the physician's ability to communicate with the patient and to understand what the patient needs. Therefore, these findings reinforce the thesis that was discussed earlier in this chapter, which holds that patient satisfaction with treatment depends both on the strictly technical as well as on the psychosocial aspects of treatment.

The physician's own satisfaction with practice must not be overlooked as a potential incentive. Beyond the financial rewards that a physician may reap from a successful practice, even beyond the satisfaction that comes from achieving and using excellent technical skills, physicians have the opportunity to improve the quality of their own work life by counselling and guiding their patients toward minimizing the impact of disease and enhancing the quality of in their lives. The ability to do this well used to be called the "art" of medicine, and the skill was never taught in medical school. Medical literature is now beginning to suggest that attention to the psychosocial aspects of patient care can have a strong positive impact on a patient's recovery.[8]

This incentive, as well as a number of others discussed in this chapter, have impelled the medical profession to examine the socialization process that has traditionally prepared physicians for practice. One result of this analysis has been the current trend to expand medical school curricula to include the teaching and practicing of interpersonal skills and the exposition of the principles of disease prevention and health promotion. As more graduates of such programs begin to practice and as the physicians who are already health promotion advocates become more visible both to their patients and their colleagues, the guidelines and examples in this book will lose their relevance.

Until then, however, educators in search of physician support will need to remember that "there are two principle influences on how physicians work: how they are trained and how they are paid."[10] At first glance, this thesis may not seem to leave much room for educators to influence physician behavior; and this may indeed be the case more often than educators and hospitals will like. However, as this chapter suggests, changing economic pressures may come to play on the side of health promotion. And finally, physicians' training to always seek the patient's good may become the best incentive for active and visible support.

References

1. Mumford, E., and others. The effects of psychological intervention on recovery from surgery and heart attacks: an analysis of the literature. American Journal of Public Health. 72:141-151, Feb. 1982.

2. Morisky, D., and others. Five-year blood pressure control and mortality following health education for hypertensive patients. American Journal of Public Health. 73:153-162, Feb. 1983.

3. Wechsler, H. and others. The physician's role in health promotion--a survey of primary care practitioners. The New England Journal of Medicine. 308:97-100, Jan. 13, 1983.

4. Press, I. A challenge for risk management. Presentation to American Society for Hospital Risk Management. 1981 Annual Meeting, Orlando, FL.

5. The effects of psychological intervention.

6. Wheat, R. P. Oh, yes, Dr. Smith: the eyes of business are upon you. Hospital Medical Staff. 11:17-21, Dec. 1982.

7. Wartman, S. A., and others. Do prescriptions adversely affect doctor-patient interactions? American Journal of Public Health. 71:1358-1361, Dec. 1981.

8. Wartman, S. and others. Impact of divergent evaluations by physicians and patients of patients' complaints. Public Health Reports. 98:141-145, March-April 1983.

9. Engel, G. The need for a new medical model: a challenge for biomedicine. Science. 196:129, 1977.

10. Jonas, S. Health-oriented physician education. Preventive Medicine. 10:700-709. 1981.

Chapter 4

THE INTERNAL AND EXTERNAL ENVIRONMENT: ITS IMPACT ON
EFFECTING CHANGE IN HEALTH PROMOTION PROGRAMS

As the previous chapters suggest, winning physicians' support for health promotion programs is rarely just a matter between a hospital's medical staff and its educators. In making patient care decisions, individual physicians will of course be influenced by some combination of incentives and disincentives that are described in Chapters 2 and 3. The individual educator will likewise behave according to a set of personal attitudes and professional habits that have been established through training and experience. Beyond these influences, however, will be another set of factors that will often have a powerful impact on the way both of these professionals behave and respond to change--an impact that neither of them, singly, will have much power to reverse.

These influences will generally be imposed by the three larger universes to which each of these professionals belongs: first, the group of colleagues (that is, the medical staff, the education department, often the nursing staff, etc.); then, the internal environment--the hospital or other institution in which these individuals work and interact; and, finally, the external environment--the immediate community that the institution serves and in which the physicians practice, as well as the wider environment that imposes economic and regulatory pressures on both. Educators who take the time to analyze how these three spheres of influence color the attitudes and behavior of the physicians--indeed, of all the relevant work groups in their institution--should be better able to work effectively within the limits that these influences impose.

Many questions need to be asked in a thorough organizational/environmental assessment, but educators should not let this be a discouragement. First of all, it is an essential first step, and the quality of the answers will help shape the department's relationship with the medical staff. Secondly, many of the answers have probably been collected by some other organizational unit in the hospital, so educators can avoid reinventing the wheel. For example, many more hospitals are now establishing a marketing function. Because the physicians in a community are primary consumers of a hospital's services, a hospital's marketing group should already have collected at least some basic information about the physicians it wishes to attract to the hospital. In addition, such information is normally collected by hospital planning departments, and some of it should also be available from departments of finance. Each of these organizational units should also be able to advise hospital-based educators about the relevant environmental questions that influence the hospital's operation and planning. Such input will offer educators the wider perspective of institution-wide goals; it will help to clarify for the educator the points of power for change and the direction in which it flows; and it will help to construct a realistic plan for engaging physicians in supporting and participating in health promotion programs.

The Characteristics of the Group

The influence exerted by a professional's immediate peer group is often a
strong one. The more established this peer group is within a particular work
environment, the less likely will be its enthusiasm for change, especially if
this change does not promise immediate and significant benefit. This principle
of individual and group behavior can be seen to apply in all the work groups
within an institution, whether they be physicians, nurses, administrators, or
others. The degree to which this behavior is apparent is often closely
related to the age of most members in a group. For example, physicians who
completed their training some time ago are unlikely to have been exposed to
the principles of health promotion in medical school to the same degree that
more recent graduates may have been. So the age of most physicians on the
medical staff--the time they have had to establish habits of practice--will
often be one indicator of their potential interest in health promotion.
However, this indicator is far from conclusive and should never be used to
stereotype an older physician group as automatic antagonists. Though younger
physicians are sometimes more likely to have been exposed to the principles of
health promotion in medical school, older physicians have been exposed to more
opportunities to put those principles into effect. If they have taken
advantage of these and seen their patients benefit from their interventions,
more experienced physicians may be strong advocates of health promotion. In
addition, it is possible that younger physicians demonstrate an interest in
health promotion not because their training has influenced them to do so, but
because an interest in wellness is popular among younger persons, especially
in some parts of the country and among certain socioeconomic groups. This
cohort effect may therefore be quickly diminished once an inexperienced
physician joins a medical staff that does not generally support health
promotion.

Another factor that will influence medical staff attitudes is the mix of
specialties that practice within the hospital. Obviously, some areas of
medical care--such as pediatrics, for example--have a longer history of
integrating some degree of patient education into their treatment approaches.
Others--such as family practice--are themselves more recent forms of organized
medical care; however, this specialty in particular has already begun to
recommend the addition of health promotion to the patient care regimens of
current practitioners by discussing these issues in their literature, The
Journal of Family Practice being one of these.

The ability of a particular specialty group to attract patients to the
hospital may be another sign of how receptive that medical staff group may be
to invitations that they support health promotion. In some instances,
physicians may consider the expansion of some hospital services--health
promotion among them--to their patient group as a device that will help them
to broaden their practice base. For example, the addition or improvement of
childbirth education may help the obstetrics/gynecology service to increase
its falling utilization rates.

The cohesiveness of the medical staff is an indicator of how likely a medical
staff is to respond in a unified fashion to any possibility of change.
Obviously, the more cohesive the group, the more predictable will be its

behavior as a group in either supporting or rejecting specific programs. Its cohesiveness will in turn be influenced by several other factors: the size of the medical staff; the presence of strong leaders and opinion-formers in the group; the extent to which medical staff members have established themselves as individual practitioners or as members of a group practice; and the level of competition that they feel with one another both in their practices in the community and in their ability to acquire various resources in the hospital.

Medical staff size will also be an influence on other characteristics. For example, if a medical staff is operating in a medium-sized hospital and has a tradition of active committee work, it may at first be difficult to identify even one or two physicians who will be willing to act as medical advisors or committee members for health promotion; most of them may already feel that they are doing more than their share.

The Characteristics of the Institution

Size will of course have an important impact on the way an entire institution operates and on its ability to respond to change. A larger institution will tend to have a more formalized organizational structure; this will also be true of its medical staff. Therefore, the decision-making about most proposed changes—especially those that would affect more than one department's functioning—will take a more complex route and will involve more participants.

The decision-making chain may become further complicated if a hospital is a teaching institution or is affiliated with a teaching institution. In such instances, an additional overlay of academic committees will tend to impose their interests on many proposals for change. Although it may take time, the health promotion function eventually may become well supported, because teaching institutions often embrace innovations that will make their patient care procedures and technologies comply with the state of the art. In comparison, smaller institutions with less bureaucratic structures may be ready to implement innovations more quickly, once the decision to accept them has been made. Another factor that tends to operate in teaching institutions more than in community hospitals is that more health professionals are involved in caring for one patient. Therefore, physicians in teaching institutions may be more used to sharing patient care responsibilities with other providers. In contrast, the community hospital environment may tend to perpetuate the more exclusionary, private relationship between one physician and one patient.

The institution's success—as measured by its occupancy rate—may have a negative affect on its medical's staff involvement in its health promotion programs. If, for example, an occupancy rate of close to 100 percent forces physicians to admit some of their patients to other hospitals in the community, their feelings of allegiance to a hospital will be split at best. In such circumstances, it is possible that they will not support the programs of one institution as much as they might if they admitted most of their patients there. It is also likely that every hospital with which physicians are affiliated will be asking for their participation in committees and other such activities; the physicians cannot possibly have time to respond to all these requests.

The location of the education function within the organizational framework will bear directly on an educator's ability to interact with the medical staff and to influence their decision-making. In many institutions, the responsibility for developing and delivering health promotion programs--especially those in patient education--lies within the nursing service. As late as 1981, an American Hospital Association survey of 5,375 hospitals indicated that 69.4 percent of them had designated a specific department for coordinating inpatient education.[1] In 39 percent of these, the department responsible was nursing inservice, while nursing administration was responsible in another 21.1 percent. The effectiveness of this arrangement depends to a great degree on the nature of the relationship between the nurses and physicians in an institution. If the quality of their interactions is generally mistrustful or antagonistic, little physician support can be initially expected for programs that nurses propose. There may be little real basis for this mistrust in the performance of patient education by either group; often, the real cause is a lack of consensus about roles. For example, a recent survey of 47 physicians, 144 registered nurses, and 28 residents who all work in the same hospital indicated that the issue of roles and responsibilities caused more dissension among the groups than did their attitudes about the need for appropriate patient education.[2] With the question, "The physician has the responsibility to determine what information the patient is to be given," 97 percent of physicians agreed; 82 percent of the residents also agreed with this statement, but only 31 percent of the nurses agreed. On the other hand, all groups generally agreed about the importance of patient education--that "patient education is an asset in providing total patient care," for example. All three groups performed at generally the same level in answering factual questions about patient education principles; that is, they all seemed to have the same basic understanding (as shown by correct answers) and the same misconceptions (as shown by incorrect answers). For example, respondents were asked to agree or disagree with the statement, "Knowledge of a disease process significantly affects patients' compliance with the treatment." Although research demonstrates that the statement is not true, only a small proporation of each group disagreed with it--11 percent of attendings, 4 percent of residents, and 6 percent of registered nurses. A survey such as this one can help to identify where the problems lie. Without an understanding of the relationships among physicians and others who are expected to perform the patient education function, an educator could waste a great deal of time designing the "perfect program" and still have it fail.

Once the basis for the relationship is clear, the educator needs to assess how a proposed program may demand that the relationship between physicians and nurses change. For example, a tradition of cooperation between the two groups may be threatened if the new program asks nurses to assume more responsibility than either they or the physician think is appropriate. Therefore, new programs that will require a drastic change in their usual roles will most probably take a longer time to become established, it they are established at all.

Some institutions have located the health promotion function in a separate department. This arrangement has both its advantages and disadvantages. On the positive side is the apparent ability this arrangement offers for the department to develop an institution-wide perspective, because it holds no inherent allegiance to any particular professional interest group. At the same time, this absence of a "connection" may be a disadvantage to the health promotion function, which could benefit from a formal tie to an established source of power and decision-making. For example, in some institutions, (such as Mercy Medical Center, Denver, CO, and St. Vincent's Hospital, Portland, OR) the health promotion function is coordinated by the same department that provides support for continuing medical education. Physicians are therefore more familiar with the education staff and may be more easily involved in program planning, development, and delivery.

Another institutional characteristic that will have a major influence on physician support for health promotion programs is the institution's formal and informal relationships with its medical staff. One good measure of this relationship is the degree to which the physicians' personal, professional, and economic goals are congruent with the goals of the institution. Other things being equal, this congruence tends to be greater as the formal ties between--and therefore the mutual interests of--physicians and hospitals increase. For example, if a group practice is directly affiliated with an institution, its physician members are more likely to foresee some benefit to themselves from supporting a new wellness center that the hospital proposes to open. If these same physicians operated a group practice that was independent of the hospital, their perception might be markedly different. Similarly, if the majority of the medical staff is related to the hospital only as admitting physicians, their commitment to institutional goals may be less than among physicians who have other roles with the institution--as salaried staff, for example, as teachers in a residency program, or as tenants in a hospital-operated medical office building.

In addition to such formal arrangements, the institution's overall stance towards the physicians who practice in the facility will generally flavor their response to suggestions of new programs. This stance is manifest in a variety of ways: the hospital's willingness to provide physicians with office support and related services; the hospital board's receptiveness to physician input--in particular, the board's willingness to accept physicians as voting members; the hospital's flexibility or rigidity in applying or modifying various relevant policies; and generally, the hospital's intent to make the institution as attractive as possible an environment in which physicians can practice. All these variables constitute a basis for physicians' future response to proposals that emanate from the hospital through its individual departments; they also influence whether a hospital and its medical staff face the external environment as separate antagonists or as a unified force with shared objectives.

The Characteristics of the External Environment

The community and the larger environment to which the hospital and its physician group offer their services constitute the largest unit in the system that educators must consider before they attempt to plan health promotion programs. This external environment will be influential in a variety of ways. For example, if several institutions provide services to the same community and compete with one another to attract admissions from the same physician group, the institutions may not wish to exert any pressure on physicians to participate in or support programs. On the other hand, if physicians have already expressed an interest in particular programs, the hospitals that best respond to that interest will be in a good position to attract those physicians and their patients (see Case 2 for a discussion of physicians' survey examples). The reverse of this situation--many physicians but few hospitals--may tend to put the institutions under less pressure and permit them to offer programs that are most in line with institutional objectives.

As was mentioned in earlier chapters, the economic environment--and specifically, changing reimbursement arrangements--can also have a major effect on physicians' support of hospital-sponsored health promotion programs. When resources to pay for patient care shrink by design of government and other third-party payers, when particular groups of patients lose their third-party coverage through unemployment, institutions and physician groups will tend to seek arrangements that promise to stabilize their economic positions. Their previous relationship with one another will often be the basis for their current response to the instability of the environment. For example, a hospital that has had mutually benefitial relationships with its medical staff may choose to join with those physicians in offering some kind of prepaid health care package to local businesses; the economic base of both parties can solidified by such an arrangement. In contrast, a previously unfriendly relationship may cause each party to seek separate, and possibly competing, solutions. The capacity of hospitals and their medical staff to consolidate their interests in such situations may provide the health promotion function with opportunities to devise new programs and expand established ones as a way of attracting individual and institutional buyers of services. On the other hand, at a time when the external environment is unfriendly to the institution and the medical staff, it is possible that the relationship between these two protagonists will be changing in some way. If the many issues they must resolve during such a time are so complex as to cause friction, the introduction of a new health promotion program may be ill-timed.

Finally, the community's need and interest in health promotion programs should play a major role both in educators' and in physicians' decision-making related to those programs. Particularly in an institution that has established formal mechanisms for community input, such as a community advisory board, the hospital will tend to be more attentive to the expressed needs of the community than it would be if no mechanism existed for gauging opinions regarding its services. To the extent that other environmental constraints permit, institutions and physicians who serve a vocal patient population will attempt to respond not only to the needs that the providers have identified but also to the needs that the community has expressed. Health promotion programs will often be included in one or both of these categories.

Having identified the major characteristics of their internal and external environment, as well as of the medical staffs whose support they seek, educators will then need to define their objectives--to choose the categories of programs that can be planned and implemented first and to decide if and how physicians may wish to be involved in the various phases of program development. Part II of this volume describes numerous successful examples of organizing physician input into and support of health promotion programs. The final chapter in Part II suggests how an understanding of physicians' attitudes toward health promotion, combined with a realistic assessment of the institutional environment, can help the educator to take the most practical and promising steps toward involving physicians in health promotion.

References

1. American Hospital Association. Special Survey on Selected Hospital Topics for 1981. Chicago: the Association, 1982.

2. Olive, D. Presentation at the Invitational Conference, "The Role of Academic Medicine in Patient Education." Sponsored by the New York Academy of Medicine, June 6 and 7, Tarrytown, NY.

PART II

SUCCESSFUL APPROACHES TO INVOLVING
PHYSICIANS IN HEALTH PROMOTION PROGRAMS

Chapter 5

BUILDING ALLIANCES OF SUPPORT

Anyone who has ever started and managed a successful program can probably recall following three rules very closely. The first is to find out if there is a need for the program and if the potential users know they need it. A second is to find at least one advocate for the program who enjoys the trust and respect of those users. And a third is to tell the potential user group about the program's benefits and qualities, in as many different ways as is appropriate, until the program's services become an accepted part of their practice. To be successful, health promotion programs must also be developed according to these rules; and because physicians are the gateway to which individuals may enter many of these programs, educators may find it valuable to think of physicians as a "user group" and to consider their needs in somewhat the same way as they do those of patients, industrial clients of employee health programs, or the community at large.

Establishing a Basis for Mutual Benefit

Asking physicians what kind of programs they believe their patients need from the health promotion staff is important in itself, so that services and needs are matched. Asking for physicians' input is also valuable in another respect; it demonstrates to them that their opinion is respected and will help to shape the programs that will eventually be offered. Experience has shown that physicians are more likely to become frequent, consistent users of programs that have been developed to suit their expressed needs. As Ted Warren, Ph.D., director of the division of education, Stormont-Vail Regional Medical Center (Topeka, KS), puts it in describing his staff's relationship with physicians, "Some programs, in areas of felt needs on the part of the medical staff, are strongly supported at any given time, while others are not supported because they are low priority needs, or not felt. The strategy we have always used in new areas of activity is to start with felt needs, do a marvelous job, and enlarge our efforts as new needs emerge."[1]

Physicians' needs for and interest in various kinds of health promotion programming can be identified in several ways; the choice depends in part on a health promotion staff's time and resources.

. At El Camino Hospital (Mountain View, CA), the director of the hospital's employee health services (called Health Management Services) and the program's medical adviser have luncheon meetings with different physicians as often as possible. This context tends to be more relaxed than an office appointment, allowing exchange to occur to the advantage of both parties. While the educator can describe the general goals of the program or the specifics of a new component, a major purpose of the meeting is to ask the physician to identify needs and interests and possibly discuss misgivings. Other program coordinators have discovered that breakfast meetings are also useful for this purpose, especially if they are trying to avoid physician's busy afternoon office hours. The early morning, before some physicians visit their hospitalized patients, seems to be a convenient time.

- If a department believes that results of a survey it conducts may not have enough credibility to influence the medical staff, using the services of a research firm to conduct a formal study may be an effective alternative. At Baptist Memorial Hospital (Memphis, TN), a firm was hired to evaluate the possible demand for a cardiac rehabilitation program. In addition to analyzing relevant characteristics of the hospital's patient population, the firm also interviewed physicians and discovered their keen interest in such a program, if it met certain criteria.

- Instead of predicting potential support for a particular program that a department is already considering, as the above strategy suggests, another kind of survey can assess the needs of the medical staff by asking for their suggestions for programs. A yearly survey sent to each physician and nurse at Decatur Memorial Hospital (Decatur, IL) asks them to suggest three patient education programs that would most benefit their patients. The results of the survey are used by the patient education advisory committee to plan programs for the following year. When the patient education department was first formed at the Day Kimball Hospital (Putnam, CT), its coordinator surveyed physicians not only on the hospital staff but also practicing in the community to discover which groups of patients were most in need of education services. The hospital's diabetes and cardiovascular teaching programs were established to respond to the priorities that survey identified.

- Less formal survey methods can be just as informative. For example, the physician chief of patient education and the department director meet periodically with the chiefs (medical directors) of other departments at Kaiser-Permanente Medical Center (Oakland, CA) to discuss the needs of those departments for new or modified programs in patient education/health promotion. This kind of interchange is expected and encouraged by the institution, which is a health maintenance organization with an institutional policy that emphasizes preventive medicine. Meetings between the department director, the physician-chief, and the chiefs of other departments are instrumental in

nurturing institution-wide support for the center's
health education programs, which include patient
education, health promotion, and other health
information services.

If the needs expressed in physician surveys are reasonable and can be filled,
programs to meet them should be developed--with care, of course, but also with
some dispatch. Especially if the health promotion department is looking for
its first "success" to change the opinions of some physicians who are not yet
supporters, a prompt response to a request or to interest expressed by those
physicians may effectively turn the tide of medical staff opinion. Case 2
offers some guidelines for conducting surveys and for using the information
they provide.

Another important tool that should not be overlooked for demonstrating
educational needs to physicians is the patient survey/satisfaction
questionnaire. Physicians are generally very interested in and sensitive to
their patients' opinions, so patients' support of a health promotion program
tends to have considerable influence with the medical staff. If a department
conducts surveys either before programs are developed or after patients have
participated in the programs, the results can be shared with the medical staff
as yet another indicator of the benefits that may accrue from well-conceived
and well-developed programming. A hospital's quality assurance mechanism can
be used to good effect in disseminating patient satisfaction information; Case
1 describes this process in more detail.

Communicating

Establishing consistent avenues of communicating survey and other program
information to the medical staff is an essential element in building physician
support. Several avenues for communicating information are generally
available in a hospital, and these can often accommodate material from the
health promotion department. If these are not adequate or accessible, new
methods can be devised. For example:

- As the previous strategies developed at Kaiser
  Permanente (Oakland, CA) suggest, the patient education
  chief is responsible for not only representing the
  department to the medical staff but also routinely
  passing on information about programs, schedules,
  materials, and so forth. At Montefiore Hospital and
  Medical Center (Bronx, NY), the chairman of the medical
  board takes on this role by regularly announcing or
  discussing patient education department developments at
  medical staff meetings.

- Existing communication tools include inhouse
  publications, such as medical staff newsletters (where
  the patient education department of Bryan Memorial
  Hospital, Lincoln, NE, publishes relevant reports and
  articles); quarterly or other periodical physicians'
  journals (such as the one published at East Tennessee

Children's Hospital, Knoxville, TN, which now routinely
publishes articles developed by the child life
coordinator and health educators on her staff); and
progress reports or even letters to the medical staff
or to physicians' offices, to announce new offerings,
program changes, or other information. When
participants in childbirth education classes at St.
Vincent Wellness Centers (Indianapolis, IN) fill out
evaluation questionnaires, the results are compiled and
reports are routinely sent to obstetricians in the
community who have referred their patients to the
classes. Joy Lomax Martin, patient education
coordinator at Baptist Memorial Hospital (Memphis, TN),
cautions that a constant onslaught of news from the
department may fall on deaf ears.[2] "We have had some
success," she reports, "by using a 'classified ad'
format in our newsletter, with the topic of the
information obviously listed at the beginning of each
section. This way, the doctor who is interested in
orthopedics will not feel obligated to read the section
on oncology support groups."

- Opportunities for two-way communication should also be
  tapped, if a relevant issue arises. One patient
  education winner of a 1982 AHA Center for Health
  Promotion Leaders Award made a point of publicizing the
  national recognition the department had won throughout
  the hospital. The result was new respect from the
  medical staff, which extended her an uncharacteristic
  invitation to make a presentation to them about the
  award-winning program. At Montefiore Hospital (Bronx,
  NY), the services of the patient education department
  are regularly discussed during grand rounds or
  specialty rounds, while at St. Vincent's Hospital
  (Portland, OR), the department of education has
  presented at two grand rounds conferences on its
  community health education programs in smoking
  cessation and weight control. (See Case 1 for further
  information.) Departmental meetings are sometimes more
  appropriate for discussing a specific program proposal
  with a physician group. If a program is aimed at a
  particular patient population, such as a cardiac
  rehabilitation program, it makes sense to direct the
  most effort to discussing it with the physicians whose
  patients would be using it most. If the wider
  community of physicians must be reached, their medical
  society meetings or their organizations' publications
  might be open to input from a local hospital's health
  promotion department.

- Even if a medical staff is generally supportive, its
  members cannot be expected to routinely orient new
  physicians to the programs and services of a health

promotion department. At Ingham Medical Center
(Lansing, MI), the patient education staff has
developed a manual as well as accompanying materials to
help new medical staff members better use the
department's services. At Montefiore Hospital (Bronx,
NY), this same objective is accomplished through an
"open house" that the patient education staff hosts
periodically for all new hospital staff members who
might use the department's services.

One major objective, of course, of communicating information about health
promotion services to physicians in the hospital and in the community is to
persuade them to refer their patients to use those services. However, unless
the message the physicians hear is credible and promising, no amount of
"media-blitz" will convince them to support the program. According to John
Mullin, director of exercise physiology services at Madison (WI) General
Hospital, "The key is to formulate complete, creative proposals for programs,
get these proposals on the agenda of appropriate medical staff section
meetings, and present the proposals for that body's consideration. Answer the
question--how can the proposed program benefit their practice in the
community?"[3]

Tapping Existing Sources of Influence

In trying to get physician support for health promotion, enough cannot be said
for the value of an influential and committed physician-advocate. This is
just as true when the purpose of the promotion is to change physicians'
patterns of health promotion as it is when a patient's health-related habits
need modification. It also tends to be true that a formal relationship with
an advocate can achieve more benefit for a program than can an informal
relationship. These two facts combined suggest two other strategies in
developing support among members of the medical staff.

The first is to identify at least one physician on the medical staff who is
already committed to the principles of health promotion and who also enjoys
the respect of colleagues. The chief of the medical staff may be a good
source of information about the interests of other medical staff members.
Medical directors of clinical departments--especially those that tend to
incorporate preventive care into their practice (e.g., family practice,
pediatrics, orthopedics, and cardiology)--may also be able to identify some
physicians who could informally guide the health promotion staff through
dealings with other physicians. A director of health promotion who is new to
a hospital may also depend on the advice of other individuals to help identify
potential physician-advocates--a predecessor in the department or its other
staff members; someone on the administrative staff who is responsible for
overseeing the health promotion department; or a nurse supervisor who has
frequent dealings with medical staff members and may be especially familiar
with their attitudes on patient education in particular as well as on other
health promotion programs.

Although it helps to have a formal relationship with a physician-advocate, the strength of an advocate's position on the medical staff may make a formal arrangement unnecessary. For example, at Madison (WI) General Hospital, the institution's medical director, a strong proponent of health promotion, was able to use his knowledge of the medical staff's keen interest in developing a cardiac surgery program to win the physicians' support for a fitness center that would also include cardiac rehabilitation facilities.

In addition to the endorsement of influential members of the medical staff (especially those in medico-administrative roles, such as the director of medical education or the vice president of medical affairs), a health promotion department should also seek the active and vocal support of the chief executive officer, appropriate members of the executive staff, and members of the board of trustees. At Appleton Memorial Hospital (Appleton, WI), the CEO has become a valuable advocate by discussing the importance of health promotion with physicians when the occasion arises. At Group Health Cooperative of Puget Sound (GHC) (Seattle, WA) it was the board of trustees that initiated the institution's new emphasis on health promotion and has been actively involved in developing the GHC's Center for Health Promotion. In many institutions, the board of trustees is not involved in making management decisions of this kind, but does establish a corporate policy to create a new kind of service that is directly responsible to the governing body; for example, the president of Health Strategies, Inc., is a physician and he reports directly to the board of this employee health service, which is affiliated with Wesley Medical Center (Wichita, KS). The board of directors of the Carl and Emily Weller Center for Health Education (Easton, PA) includes several spouses of physicians, who have been very valuable advocates in gaining physician support for this center's programs in community health promotion.

The support of a local medical society may also be helpful, especially if many physicians in the hospital belong to it and if its programs and services are useful to them. Contacting the society directly or through one of its members should reveal the group's stance toward relevant health promotion issues. If the society takes a negative view of the hospital's initiating communitywide health promotion programs or offering employee health services to local industry, the health promotion director as well as the CEO may find it useful to establish a dialogue with the society and request to use some of its meetings as a forum for discussion and possibly for reaching some measure of agreement.

An example of positive medical society influence on physicians' support of health promotion is the Center for Health Education, Inc. (Baltimore, MD), which is a new joint venture of the Medical and Chirurgical Faculty of the State of Maryland and Blue Cross and Blue Shield of Maryland. One of its functions is to develop continuing education programs for physicians in the techniques of promoting healthy lifestyles among their patients. These programs involve physicians in training physicians; a recent course was designed to teach physicians how to encourage compliance with hypertension regimens. The presence of such strong, local advocacy groups among physicians should be a useful resource to health promotion programs in a community. A hospital-based department may wish to follow the group's agenda, help to publicize it to its own medical staff, and create opportunities for reinforcing the contents of the group's agenda through its own programs.

In addition to forming informal ties with physician-advocates, a second strategy is to engage such physicians in formal relationships with the health promotion department. Their role in its activities will help ensure the credibility of program content among their colleagues; it may also help generate other physicians' participation. A variety of structures can be established both within and outside the department by which physicians' consistent input into health promotion programs can be organized. For example:

- An individual physician can become a liaison between the department and the medical staff. At Kaiser Permanente Medical Center (Oakland, CA) a physician chief of patient education shares with the medical center's administrator the responsibility of supervising the director of health education. A position that imposes less direct management responsibility may be created by appointing a medical advisor to the department of health education.

- Because a close interaction is often required between an occupational health service and its users' sources of medical care, establishing a formal position for a medical director of occupational health services appears to be a very effective means for initiating and maintaining communications with these providers. This experience has been reported by several institutions, including St. Joseph's Hospital (Omaha, NE), and Duke University Medical Center (Durham, NC); similarly, at Paoli Hospital (Paoli, PA), a committee on occupational health was able to function more effectively when its chairmanship was assumed by a physician.

- Physicians may become involved in health promotion activities at a hospital by becoming active members of a variety of committees. At Decatur Memorial Hospital (Decatur, IL), a patient education committee, which includes two physicians in its multidisciplinary membership, meets monthly to deliberate policies, programs, resources, and other issues relevant to patient education programming. In addition, all members are responsible for communicating information concerning patient education activities and programs to the specific groups they represent.

- Some physicians may be reluctant to take on a long-term appointment either as medical director or as a member of a committee that deals with overall health promotion activities at their hospital. However, they may be very willing to participate in an ad hoc committee or a standing committee created to deal with issues that relate to one of their special clinical interests. At Kaiser Permanente (Oakland, CA), this kind of opportunity is available through such committees as the cancer education committee and the pre-op teaching

committee. The community health education program at
United General Hospital (Sedro Wolley, WA) invited five
physicians and their spouses to join a panel to
evaluate the program only five months after its
inception. Their review formed the basis for program
revision and helped to encourage the shift of physician
opinion from scepticism to support.

An institution where all of these structures are used to ensure physician
involvement is the Group Health Cooperative (GHC) of Puget Sound (Seattle, WA),
a health maintenance organization that owns two hospitals, three specialty care
centers, and 12 primary care medical centers. In the mid-1970s, the
all-consumer governing board of this organization decided to place a stronger
emphasis on health promotion. One way it chose to do so was by greatly
expanding the staff and the budget for health education activities. However,
the board received minimal physician input into either the boards'
deliberations on the issues nor into the development of the new service.
Because the physicians are employees of the cooperative, says George A. Orr
III, director of the GHC's Center for Health Promotion (CHP), they have a
bigger stake in what services are provided and they also expect to have a
proportionate share of influence and control over those services.[4] The
confrontation that followed the board's unilateral decision was resolved only
after considerable negotiation, which resulted in some formal structures being
developed for physician input into health education program development and
management processes. For example, a quarter-time medical staff director
position was established with responsibilities for setting priorities for new
patient education programs, with the input of a multidisciplinary patient
education steering committee that the physician co-chairs with the CHP staff
coordinator. (See p. 41 for full statement of medical staff director
responsibilities.) "The physicians do much of the patient education here,"
says Orr, "and the education staff's role is to back them up, so it makes
sense that they should set the priorities." In turn, the CHP staff defines
the most appropriate educational methods for each program.

As a need for a program is identified in the area of patient education or
preventive medicine, which has a separate medical staff director, a physician
advisor is assigned to that program, to work with its program coordinator and
to act as an additional liaison to the medical staff. In comparison to the
friction that marked their earlier relationship, reports Orr, the GHC Center
for Health Promotion benefits considerably from the "collegial relationship"
that now exists with the medical staff. As this example clearly demonstrates,
formalizing the tie between a department and its physician-advocates can
greatly enhance the value of the relationship. If the responsibility of
assisting in planning and consulting on medical content of programs is defined
in a medical advisor's/medical director's statement of responsibilities, the
department can depend on a consistent source of medical input and a route for
access to the rest of the medical staff.

References

1. Warren, T., Ph.D. Personal communication, Feb. 1, 1983.

2. Martin, J. Personal communication, Dec. 22, 1982.

3. Mullin, J. Personal communication, Jan. 14, 1983.

4. Orr, G. III. Personal communication, May 10, 1983.

Group Health Cooperative of Puget
  Sound, Seattle, WA

JOB RESPONSIBILITY
STATEMENT

TITLE: MEDICAL STAFF DIRECTOR OF PATIENT EDUCATION

REPORTS TO: Medical Director

OVERALL
RESPONSIBILITY: To assure the assessment of needs and the determination of
                program directions and priorities for the patient education
                activities of the Center for Health Promotion (CHP). To be
                jointly responsible for patient education program budget
                development and program evaluation with the Director of
                Health Promotion.

PERFORMANCE
APPRAISAL: The incumbent's effectiveness in carrying out the duties
                specified in this job description will be evaluated by the
                Medical Director.

SPECIFIC RESPONSIBILITIES:

Patient Education Program Development

- Assess, with the assistance of the CHP Staff, needs for patient
  education. This will be done with the input of providers, consumers,
  and management.

- Determine topic areas for patient education based on needs assessments.

- Prioritize program directions (topic areas) for CHP patient education
  activities based on needs assessment.

- Assist the CHP in developing specific patient education programs in
  the capacity of planner/consultant.

- Assure that the medical content of patient education materials and
  curricula is accurate and current.

Communications

- Establish and maintain positive communications between the CHP and the
  medical staff in order to:

  1) communicate medical staff needs, priorities, and concerns to the
     CHP.

  2) communicate information on patient education programs and
     priorities at GHC to the medical staff.

3) maintain the credibility of the CHP within the medical staff.

4) resolve intra-medical staff conflicts about the priorities, content, and educational methodologies of CHP patient education activities.

Budget

. Be jointly responsible with the Director of Health Promotion for determining budgetary needs for the patient education activities of the department.

Coordination

. Take a leadership role, in concert with the CHP staff, to coordinate the CHP's patient education program with the patient education programs of other GHC departments. The intent will be to increase the overall educational impact by focusing on common goals.

Evaluation

. Jointly assess, with the Director of Health Promotion, the impact of CHP patient education programs.

Miscellaneous

. Provides consultation to the CHP on issues and programs related to prevention and wellness.

. Chair the GHC Patient Education Steering Committee.

9/4/81 Update of description as contained in Medical Staff Rules & Regulations, August, 1980.

Chapter 6

INVOLVING PHYSICIANS IN PROGRAM DEVELOPMENT

The best reason for making good planning a part of any product development
process is to ensure that the product will be not only useful but also used.
This is also the best reason for encouraging physician involvement in the
planning of health promotion programs. Unless physicians approve of the text
of teaching materials distributed to their cardiac patients, unless they
believe the programs of a fitness center have a sound medical basis--in
general, unless the content and benefits of a given program meet physicians'
standards, they will most probably not refer patients to the program. To
avoid this situation, educators must elicit the input of their own medical
staff members at several points in the process of program development.

The fact that input must come from the physicians who use that institution--
rather than from some other individual physician or group--cannot be stressed
enough. Programs developed elsewhere, with the preferences of other
physicians in mind, will often contain elements inconsistent with a given
medical staff's philosophy or methodology. In certain cases, such programs
may be as unacceptable to some members of a medical staff as would be programs
with no physician input whatsoever. This may be especially true if competition
is strong between two medical staffs from institutions in the same community
or within the same multihospital arrangement. There are exceptions to this
general rule, of course. If widely-respected physicians from their own peer
group have helped to develop a program, it will probably make less difference
that they are not from the same institution. Likewise, materials developed by
medical associations, such as the American Medical Association's Patient
Medication Information sheets, should also be widely accepted.

Physicians should be able to choose from a variety of ways to join in the
process of program planning and development--either through direct
participation in the organizational unit that is responsible for developing a
program; through membership in medical staff committees with some
responsibility for health promotion activities, or as individual medical staff
members.

Input from the Department's Physician Associates

The most logical source of medical input into program planning is the physician
or physicians who have already committed themselves to some formal
relationship with the health promotion department.

  - The first of these should be the department's medical
    director. As the examples in Chapter 5 suggest, a
    physician in this role can help in all aspects of
    planning. At the Group Health Cooperative of Puget
    Sound (Seattle, WA), the medical staff director of
    patient education has responsibilities for program

planning clearly defined in a "job responsibility statement" (see Chapter 5 for more information). In addition to prioritizing the content areas in which programs are to be developed, the medical staff director must "assist....in developing specific patient education programs in the capacity of planner/consultant" and "assure that the medical content of patient education materials and curricula is accurate and current." Helping to evaluate the impact of these programs and to coordinate them with the programs of other departments are also part of this director's responsibilities.

. The medical director can also help identify other physicians on the medical staff who may be willing or interested in participating in a planning effort. At El Camino Hospital (Mountain View, CA), the medical director of the health promotion program performs this role as he and the program's administrator attempt to develop support through periodic meetings with individual physicians. At the Group Health Cooperative of Puget Sound (GHC) (Seattle, WA), the process of finding other physicians to participate in program planning is more formalized. Each new program of the Center for Health Promotion has a medical staff advisor appointed by the GHC medical director, with recommendations from the medical staff director of patient education and the medical staff director of preventive care research. The programs vary from such patient education offerings as diabetes education to community health classes in fitness. According the medical staff advisor job description, the physician's responsibilities may include that of advisor in program planning, consultant on the state-of-the-art and on medical content of the program, reviewer of program materials, reviewer on other aspects of the program (such as defining program population, commenting on its practicality in primary care, etc.), and advisor for the program's quality assurance component. The statement also clarifies the responsibilities the advisor will not be expected to assume, such as being identified as the "expert" that consumers seek out on the program's content; the list of roles that the medical advisor will not be expected to play serves to protect that physician from excessive demands from GHC consumers or staff and to ensure that the panel system approach of GHC is preserved.

. Physicians who join hospital-wide patient education committees expect to participate in program planning at least to some degree. When possible, their participation should be active rather than reactive; that is, their input should begin early, as the need for a new program is identified, as the characteristerics of the target population are described, as content and appropriate methodology are developed. The multidisciplinary patient education steering committee at Mount Auburn Hospital (Cambridge, MA) includes physicians in its membership. Responsibility for the management of hospital-wide patient and family education are centralized within this committee; during its monthly meetings, it plans, coordinates inplementation of, and evaluates patient education programs, while department-level committees develop specific materials and implement those plans.

• A patient education committee at St. Mary-Rogers Memorial Hospital (Rogers, AR) plans community education activities to supplement those sponsored by the hospital's education department. Although two physicians (one of them, the chief of staff) were interested in establishing such a group for some time, it was not until a local chiropractor offered a widely publicized education program to the community that the hospital's physicians agreed that such a planning group was necessary to ensure the community's access to correct health-related information. The committee includes five physicians, the director of and one instructor from the education department, as well as several representatives from the community. One of the committee's first projects was to establish a speaker's bureau, which is coordinated by the hospital's education department and in which almost all the physicians who use the hospital are enrolled.

• The six physicians who compose the medical review committee for community wellness programs of Brackenridge Hospital (Austin, TX) are recommended for membership by the chief of the medical staff and the hospital administrator. Their primary purpose, as the title of the committee implies, is to review early drafts of program materials. Each program is offered in the form of a class, usually to groups that are associated with community organizations (such as churches) or to local employers. Each of the classes has its own workbook, and the names of the physician reviewers is listed in each workbook. An example of the kind of input physicians offer comes from the wellness staff's work in developing a workbook for a physical fitness class, during which their research suggested that an individual must always check with a physician before beginning an exercise program; a strong recommendation to this effect was therefore included in an early version of the workbook that the committee reviewed. The physicians suggested that this was too stringent a precaution and that it would

discourage too many individuals from beginning an
exercise program. The committee recommended that the
precaution be modified and made more specific to those
whose health warranted a medical check-up before they
began a fitness program. Review comments like these
have been useful in program development as well as in
program marketing. The physician's input helps to
ensure the medical soundness of the program, and this
in turn tends to assure other physicians as well as
potential program participants. The review process
itself has been designed not to encumber either the
physicians or the wellness program staff with too heavy
a committment of time for meetings: materials are
mailed to each committee member, and they may return
their comments either by mail or telephone.

. Physicians who do not have either the time for or the
interest in addressing a broad range of issues in
health promotion may be willing to join an effort that
draws on their particular specialty or interest. At
United and Children's Hospitals (St. Paul, MN), the
administration's interest in developing an occupational
health program for local industry employees was
tempered somewhat by a cautious response from those
members of the medical staff who had a vested interest
in maintaining their services to their industrial
clients. However, these physicians' stance toward the
idea was not entirely negative, in part because the
hospital permitted them to use its own employee health
service facilities to perform preemployment physical
examinations for their clients' applicants for
employment. In addition, the hospital, through one of
its vice presidents in charge of the project, clearly
expressed its intention to develop services that would
supplement those of the physicians, not compete with
them. On this basis, the 50 or so physicians who have
formal provider or consultant relationships with local
industry were willing to discuss the possibilities of
an occupational health program. They formed a
loosely-knit advisory committee, which directs its
input to the department of occupational therapy and
rehabilitation. The committee's initial task was to
define some specific needs for occupational health
services, based on the physicians' experiences with
their own clients. These will be compared to the
results of an industry market survey that the
department conducted and is preparing to present to the
committee. The comparison should then form the basis
for the committee's cooperating in planning and
developing the occupational health programs. (See Case
3 on committees.)

Input from Medical Staff Committees

The need for--and the effort of--establishing separate committees for planning and developing various programs may be eliminated if a medical staff committee already exists that can and will take on the task. The advice of the chief of the medical staff, the vice president for medical affairs, or some other physician in a similar administrative position can be invaluable to the educator who is trying to develop a physician support network. A piecemeal approach is likely to produce piecemeal results, while the use of a long standing committee structure might be an acceptable way of introducing a new program to the medical staff and generally giving some physicians a first taste of the benefits that health promotion programs might offer. Each institution has its own committee hierarchy and its own methods for adding or changing committee charges; the educator should become familiar with these and again depend on the advice and help of a physician-administrator who can better steer such a change through the process.

Once the committee charge has been passed on and accepted, a medical staff committee can provide input into all the phases of program planning.

- To begin with, a committee can help to identify the need for a program. For example, the Child Life Department at East Tennessee Children's Hospital (Knoxville, TN) was established after nine months of planning, in which both the medical executive committee (composed of the chiefs of all clinical services) and one of it subcommittee's, the medical staff committee, were active participants. The department was then established to meet the educational and recreational needs of pediatric patients and their families.

- Suggestions for program changes can also originate in medical staff committees, as they do at East Tennessee Children's. Once the Child Life Department was established, the medical-nursing liaison committee assumed an advisory role to the department. Its membership includes the hospital's administrator, the chief of medicine, the chief of surgery, the assistant administrator of patient services, the two child life coordinators, the assistant director of nursing, and a head nurse. Although the two physician chiefs are the department's primary advisors, this committee provides periodic input into department activities by both suggesting new programs and assisting in the preparation of materials.

- The medical staff education committee at Mount Auburn Hospital (Cambridge, MA) serves both as program planner and program reviewer, depending on the circumstances. For example, this committee cooperated with the patient care and ambulatory care committees to plan and develop the hospital's cardiac rehabilitation patient education program.

- Although it is wise to seek physicians' input in the early stages of program developmemt, at the very least physicians should be asked to review a program before it is implemented. An appropriate group of reviewers may be found in a medical staff committee whose responsibilities are related to the program's content. The surgical staff committee at Decatur Memorial Hospital (Decatur, IL) reviewed and approved the mastectomy rehabilitation program that was developed through a multidisciplinary effort. In comparison, Bryan Memorial Hospital, where physicians are involved in early program planning, formal channels have also been developed for their approval of all education programs; these include any appropriate physician committee and the medical staff executive committee as well as review by the hospital practice subcommittee on patient education.

- At Columbus Children's Hospital (Columbus, OH), the Homegoing Education and Literature Program (H.E.L.P.) within the nursing education department is responsible for managing the development of written patient/family education materials, which are called "Helping Hand" teaching aids. The traditional committee structure is not used in any aspect of this program, because, by consensus, all the members of the health care team are actively involved in teaching patients and families. Therefore, they all serve as members of "a committee of the whole" and all participate in developing program materials. However, because this informal "committee" is so large, the process of reviewing materials as they are developed has been highly formalized and is represented by a flow chart (See figure on following page), which stipulates physician participation at four points.

Input from Individual Physicians

As a medical staff grows larger, a smaller proportion of its physicians is involved in any particular committee. Consequently, the negative opinions of a few physicians about any given program plan may be overlooked, sometimes until it is too late to respond to those opinions without undoing or redoing a great deal of work. The educator should make the effort to identify and seek out these physicians, especially if their responses or their medical input might make or break the usefulness and the use of a new program.

- For example, at one hospital in the midwest, the medical staff of 100 or so physicians does not routinely accept invitations to participate in any patient education committee. They are not yet convinced of the need for such a committee, nor do they

Flow Chart for Developing Helping Hand Teaching Aids

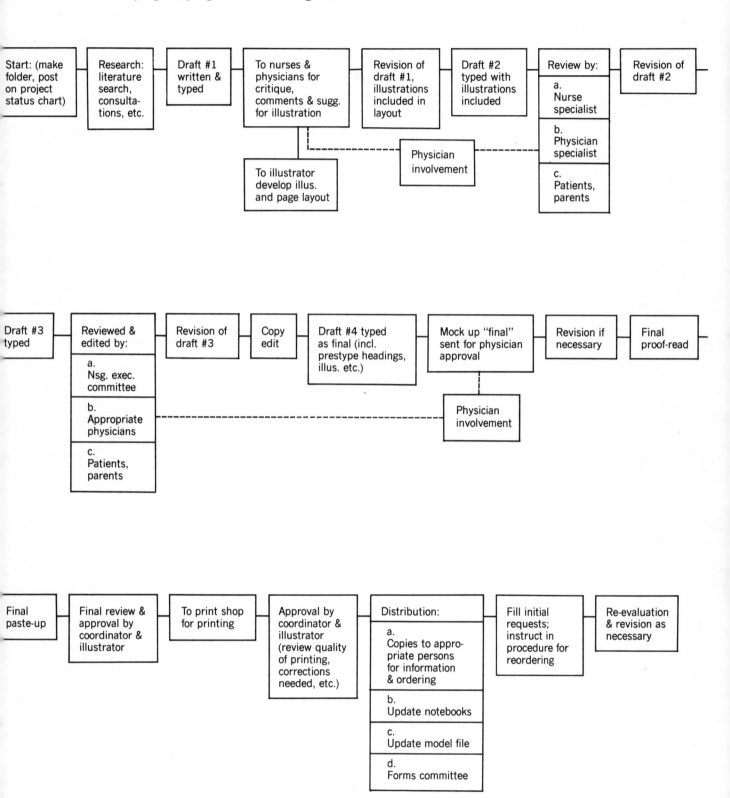

feel they have the time to commit to an effort many of
them believe is adequately taken care of in the normal
course of physician-patient communications. However,
individual physicians do respond to requests to review
programs as they are being planned and developed, as
they did with a preoperative teaching program and
another for diabetic patients. The patient education
coordinator identifies these physicians by their
specialty, by the numbers of patients they admit to the
hospital who might benefit from the program, and by
other such relevant factors. Although most of the
physicians are proponents of both programs (e.g., most
diabetic teaching is now done by nurses without a
physician's order), some key physicians are taking a
very cautious stance toward the development of a new
cardiac inpatient education program. One of the
sources of their scepticism is a long-standing friction
between what is a conservative medical staff and a
nursing staff that includes individuals who wish to
assume more responsibility in patient care--and in
patient education, in particular. This friction was
further fueled when several nurses and allied health
staff took it upon themselves to develop a cardiac
teaching program without either physician input or
final approval. The program remains unused, and the
patient education coordinator must slowly repair the
rift with physicians by ensuring that a new program
does have physician input. One nurse, whose approach
to this issue is acceptable to these physicians, has
assumed the task of developing a program that may meet
their approval.

. When a medical staff is so large or the nature of the
materials is such that individual contact with
physicians regarding every new program can be
inefficient, another strategy must be found. At the
University of Maryland Hospital (Baltimore, MD), all
patient education programs that will be implemented on
a hospital-wide basis are submitted for preliminary
review to a subcommittee of the medical board. If a
program is in an audio-visual form, it is then
displayed for several weeks in the media library so
that the entire medical staff may view it before it is
submitted for final approval.

. Finally, the most elementary strategy for involving an
individual physician in program planning is to ask for
advice on how to teach an individual patient. The
mechanism for such involvement is already established
in institutions that have a team approach to patient
care and teaching, by which a patient's physician meets
periodically with team members to develop a plan of
care. Where no such mechanisms exist, educators must

create substitutes, as a few nurses at St. John's
Hospital (Salina, KS) have done by preparing lists of
questions that patients with certain problems ask
routinely; these questions are submitted to the
patients' respective physicians, so that they may
advise the nurses how they want their patients to be
informed.

And so a beginning is made.

Chapter 7

ENCOURAGING PHYSICIANS TO PROMOTE PROGRAMS

As Part I of this volume suggests, each physician has a different set of
reasons for not involving patients in health promotion activities. Some of
these have to do with habit; some others stem from physicians not having ready
information about programs at their fingertips and not having the time to find
it. Education program planners must therefore make program marketing a
fundamental component of their efforts. The results of a needs assessment,
conducted among physicians before program planning was even begun (see Chapter
5 and Case 2 for further details), could now be used for another purpose--as
the basis for encouraging physicians' support for health promotion programs
among their patients.

Disseminating Program Information

The physician who knows where and when to send a patient for a program--be it
prenatal classes, stress reduction, or cardiovascular rehabilitation--is
several steps ahead of the physician who doesn't, and so is the patient.
Making this kind of information readily available to the medical staff is the
first part of program promotion, and it can be accomplished in many different
ways.

- At Montefiore Hospital and Medical Center (Bronx, NY),
  the patient education department uses several different
  avenues to introduce new programs and to refresh
  memories about ongoing activities. The department
  hosts an "open house" periodically, to which all the
  health professionals working in the hospital are
  invited. Department staff members use these events to
  describe new programs and resources and to elicit
  valuable feedback from those who attend. In addition,
  the hospital's deputy director of professional affairs
  (who is himself a physician) periodically mails a
  reminder to all the hospital's physicians that the
  patient education department offers a variety of
  services; the letter briefly describes these and
  emphasizes the fact that all programs and all patient
  education materials have been reviewed and approved by
  appropriate physicians. Single copies of all new
  materials developed by the department are mailed to all
  the hospital's attending physicians, who are welcome to
  order more copies to use in their offices. These
  materials are also collected in a patient education
  manual that is available for physicians' reference on
  each nursing unit, where multiple copies of these
  materials (in English and Spanish) are kept in files to
  be handed out to patients. Finally, a quarterly

newsletter for physicians describes new programs
offered by the patient education department; it lists
dates, times, and other pertinent information and
generally encourages physicians to call the department
for any support or information they may need.

- When the Cardiac Rehabilitation Team was first
established at Ingham Medical Center (Lansing, MI),
team members often found that orders written for their
involvement in a patient's rehabilitation regimen were
inconsistent with the team's established protocol. The
problem occurred most often with orders written by
physicians new to the medical staff or by new
residents. The team tried two solutions--verbal
orientation of these physicians first by the team
coordinator and then by the cardiologist who was the
team's medical advisor. When neither of these totally
eliminated the inconsistencies, the team developed a
manual that puts the protocol in writing and is made
available to all new residents, to new medical staff
members in cardiology and internal medicine, and to any
other physician who appears to have difficulty
following the protocol. The manual describes the role
of each team member (physician, CCU nurse, medical
social worker, physical therapist, occupational
therapist, cardiac rehabilitation nurse, dietician,
pharmacist, home care coordinator, and clinic nurse),
and suggests to the physician the kind of specific
information each needs to perform his or her aspect of
care. The team has found that the written protocol has
not only reduced many of the previous problems with
order writing but also seems to have increased
referrals and encouraged physicians to request the
team's involvement earlier in a patient's course of
recovery.

- Physicians who have not had the opportunity to view
audiovisual programs before they are made available to
patients through a hospital's closed circuit television
program may hesitate to suggest these programs to their
patients. Even if they have seen a program, they may
have forgotten the specific program content, and only a
title listing in a CCTV schedule does not refresh their
memories. A CCTV program schedule that briefly
describes each program as well as listing the
"show-time" can be kept at each nurses' station for
physicians' easy reference as they are writing orders.

- At Kaiser Permanente Medical Center (Oakland, CA),
physicians can carry a schedule of major patient
education offerings with them; printed in a narrow
pamphlet form, the schedule fits easily into a lab coat
pocket and lists programs, times, and patient education
staff telephone numbers to call for further information.

- At Kettering (OH) Medical Center, a telephone number is the key to patients' access to "prescription programming" on the closed circuit television system. To ensure that physicians keep this telephone number in mind, the media department has imprinted it on coffee mugs and tote bags and has distributed these to physicians who are most likely to order the "prescription programming" service for their patients.

- Any route that physicians routinely use to get to useful information is one that educators can use to pass on information about programs. For example, in a teaching hospital, medical rounds are sometimes an occasion for pharmaceutical representatives to set up displays of literature and other materials. Because physicians are accustomed to stopping and examining these, educators could consider adding a display rack of materials for their department's programs and services. Special attention could be drawn to any items that relate to a particular day's topic for rounds.

- Certainly any number of other methods may be used to give program information to physicians, although each of these should be used judiciously; a barrage of paper is seldom appreciated, and eventually, much of it is simply ignored. Periodic notices may be posted in the physicians' lounge or some other strategic point; however, it is wise to check in advance whether anyone can post such notices or if a medical staff secretary or some other person must screen them first.

- Program schedules can also be mailed to physicians' offices, and this is especially appropriate if the hospital offers outpatient education, community health education, and other wellness programs. At Decatur (IL) Memorial Hospital, a quarterly newsletter is mailed to physicians' office nurses on the premise that physicians, especially those who are new to the community, do not have the time to keep track of the health promotion offerings in a community, and so they delegate this task to their office staff. The newsletter makes the task easier by describing the new program offerings at the hospital, listing new printed education materials that are available for free to physicians' offices, and generally discussing how the nurses and other appropriate staff can help to add a health promotion dimension to the physicians' practice.

Facilitating Referrals

Once physicians have appropriate program information available, a variety of other approaches can help them routinely incorporate the information into their patient treatment options. For example:

- Members of the St. Joseph Hospital (Omaha, NE) medical staff are encouraged to give their patients with work-related health problems more than just a written medical excuse from several days of work. At medical staff meetings, through individual contact, and by word of mouth, the occupational health service (OHS) staff has attempted to convince physicians of the importance of education in helping their patients to avoid health hazards at work. The staff has also assured these physicians that its purpose is not to compete for their patients, but rather to reciprocate referrals as often as possible. When a patient is sent to the OHS by one of its business/industry clients for preemployment testing or some other such service, OHS staff always determine whether the patient has a family physician; if not, the patient is given three names of physicians (chosen by rotation from a medical staff list) and urged to establish contact with one of them. If the patient is in need of medical care at the time he applies to OHS, the staff often calls a physician's office immediately to make the appointment and to pass on relevant information. Although the OHS staff has not been able to measure the effectiveness of this strategy in terms of reciprocal referrals from physicians, Joseph Fanucchi, M.D., the department's director, feels that the OHS was able to avoid a great deal of opposition from physicians by making its reciprocal referral policy clear before it even opened its doors.[1] Another tool that Dr. Fanucchi would like to develop would be a record of all patients who have been referred to physicians in the community; he feels such a list would be clear evidence to these physicians of the OHS' intent to cooperate with them and to complement their services.

- Physicians in community practice may be convinced of the potential benefits of some of the health promotion programs a hospital offers. However, they may not have a ready technique for identifying those patients who may be appropriate candidates for specific programs. A health hazard appraisal program sponsored by the hospital could be made available to such physicians as a tool to better identify patients at risk, to help motivate these patients to reduce those risks, and as an additional service to help expand the physicians' base.[2]

- The smoking management seminars offered by Presbyterian-St. Luke's Medical Center (Denver, CO) attract physicians' referrals by giving them the chance to pass on a fee discount to any patient they refer. A special prescription pad is provided to physicians who are associated with the hospital. Along with a blank space for the patient's name and the physician's signature, the prescription announces that, "on presentation of this sheet a $50.00 reduction off tuition will be granted to the above."

. Once a physician begins to refer his office patients to health promotion programs at the hospital, the pattern should be reinforced when appropriate. For example, the patient education arm of the nursing staff development office at St. Mary's Hospital (Decatur, IL) routinely provides feedback on such referrals by sending the physician a notification of the patient's attendance, expressing thanks for the referral, and adding any other information that would be useful in medical follow-up.

. Inhouse referral patterns can also be established more easily by making some simple changes in patients' medical charts. At Kaiser Permanente Medical Center (Oakland, CA), a patient education referral slip is attached to each patient's chart to remind physicians, as they are making notes in the chart, to consider whether some form of education might be appropriate. A checklist of seven patient education and four nutrition education offerings is printed on the slip, so that all a physician needs to do is either check the appropriate box or specify some other program in the space provided. To reinforce these referrals, various departments, such as respiratory therapy, use a rubber stamp to add information to the patient's chart regarding the patient's attendance at a program and a brief description of the program's content; the stamp also provides some space for the instructor's comment, if any. The cardiac rehabilitation team at Ingham Medical Center (Lansing, MI) requested that an addition be made to the routine order sheet that initiates a patient's transfer from a critical care unit to a general medical floor; the addition simply requires physicians to check "yes" or "no" if they wish the team to become involved in a patient's continuing care. This change in the chart has encouraged physicians who are neither cardiologists nor internists to consider whether the team's services might benefit a patient whose hospitalization was precipitated by some other problem.

The point of this variety of strategies, then, is to encourage physicians to use the resources of the hospital to the fullest, so that their own efforts to inform and teach the patient may be supplemented by the organized efforts of educators in the hospital. Helping physicians refine their own teaching skills is also an important consideration in developing an overall plan for increasing physician involvement in health promotion; some examples of how this can be done are described in the following chapter.

References

1. Fanucchi, J., M.D.   Personal communication, March 1, 1983.

2. Dunton, S.   A basic introduction to the health hazard appraisal.   <u>Promoting Health</u>.   2:1-3, July-Aug. 1981.

Chapter 8

HELPING PHYSICIANS TO DO HEALTH PROMOTION

While both the physician and the patient have always considered the exchange of information to be an important part of their relationship, they have not--and do not--always agree about how successful the exchange has been. Indeed, the extent to which a physician actually passes information on to a patient for the purpose of improving the patient's health often diminished by a variety of factors, some of which are discussed in Part I of this volume. The effect is not always to the patient's benefit.

Medical care of diabetes, which afflicts more than six million Americans, is a good example. According to the National Diabetes Advisory Board, not only has significant and correct clinical information not reached the large number of health care providers who treat 80 percent of the diabetic population; the Board also considers the lack of patient education in the private practice setting to be a major barrier to effective care of diabetic patients. "Those responsible for patient education often do not have the time or the information to do the task. The third barrier identified is the lack of interaction within and among the components of the health care system. Thus with no community plan, only the motivated, better educated patients are able to utilize resources in a rational cost-effective manner."[1]

The hospital-based health educator is in an excellent position to help overcome all three of these barriers, whether they be related to diabetes or to a variety of other health problems. Certainly some of the strategies described in Chapter 7 can bring to the physician and so to the patient information about hospital-based programs that are relevant to the patient's care. It is equally important, however, to help physicians to do the teaching--and to do it better and more consistently than many of them have until now.

Helping Physicians to Develop Their Teaching Skills

Many physicians believe that their current communications with their patients already include an adequate teaching component and that any improvement would be superfluous. This is not always the case. However, these same physicians do not often attempt to relate a patient's noncompliance or lack of improvement in health status to the shortcomings in their own teaching methods. Other physicians may make the connection but not know how to overcome the problem in an organized way.

Educators can help physicians to identify the tools that are most appropriate for diagnosing and improving their teaching skills and then for putting these skills to most effective use in their practice. For example:

- A number of programs have already been developed by medical schools, medical associations, and other agencies to help physicians improve the quality of their communication with their patients. The Extended Programs in Medical Education at the University of California San Francisco School of Medicine have developed a tool called PROCAP--Professional Competence Assurance Program for Practicing Physicians.[2] One of its components is designed to help physicians evaluate their care and teaching of diabetic patients through both medical record review and a survey sent to their patients concerning their knowledge, compliance, and self-care practices related to diabetes. A report of both record and survey data is generated by a PROCAP computer and compares each physician to others in the program's sample. While maintaining the individual physician's confidentiality, the program provides each with a "diagnosis" of deficits and an individualized educational program. This includes a syllabus (with copies of patient handouts) and a conference call that links a faculty "expert" with several practitioners who have demonstrated a similar level of proficiency. Each physician also receives a community diabetes resource directory, which is prepared by the local chapter of the American Diabetes Association. Programs such as this one, and others that are listed in the appendix on resources, can be especially useful for physicians who want some evidence of their own effectiveness as teachers. It may also be an attractive alternative for those physicians who dislike attending seminars and other such events.

- Although not all physicians prefer them, organized group teaching--in seminars, workshops, and other such events--can be a very useful way to reach a large number of physicians at one time. The educator can either help organize such programs (a grand rounds, for example) or offer to supplement their content with related patient teaching materials (for example, by working with a physician who is presenting a case during a clinical department meeting). The credibility of the program's sponsors should be a good indicator of physicians' potential interest in the program--and in the patient teaching concepts and materials that it includes. The educator can get information about forthcoming programs that may offer such opportunities for cooperation from a number of sources. An inhouse medical staff publication will no doubt make such announcements. The education department's medical advisor and its physician committee members may also pass on such information, especially if the educator expresses specific interest and explains how such events may be used to promote physicians' direct involvement in patient teaching.

. A medical staff's current interest in some clinical
problem might also be a good opportunity to increase
physicians' awareness of its related health promotion
component. Even if no program has been organized to
discuss the topic, the health education staff can
provide teaching materials through a display in the
physicians' lounge and describe useful teaching methods
and tools in an inhouse publication that physicians are
likely to read. Again, the department's medical
advisor or some other knowledgeable physician can offer
clues about current topics of interest.

Donald Iverson, Ph.D., who is director of the health promotion/disease
prevention (HP/DP) program at Mercy Medical Center (Denver, CO), offers
several guidelines for developing continuing education programs (CME) for
physicians:

. "It is not unrealistic for even small institutions to
provide educational experiences for their physician
staff," Dr. Iverson suggests, "but they will have the
greatest chance for success if they use educational
mechanisms that have previously attracted the most
physician involvement--whether this is grand rounds or
CME or some other forum."[3] At Mercy Medical Center,
for example, residents and staff are invited to bring
their lunch to periodic noon-time conferences, where a
physician from the teaching staff and a health educator
discuss the disease prevention and health promotion
aspects of a particular condition. At a recent
conference, which was attended not only by residents
but also by staff from nursing, physical therapy, and
some other departments, the topic was the
identification of patients at risk for low back pain.
Using a live model, the physician described techniques
to be used during a physical exam and the educator
demonstrated exercises to be taught to patients who are
at risk or suffer from low back pain. Conference
participants received printed materials that repeated
and reinforced the information they had heard.

. None of the techniques or interventions recommended
during this conference would have taken a physician
much time to complete during a routine medical
encounter. This point was emphasized several times
during the conference and is another guideline to
remember. "Whatever these programs attempt to teach
physicians to do," Dr. Iverson says, "they should keep
in mind the constraints of a physician's practice.
Therefore the protocol that is recommended must be easy
to do, easy to incorporate in an office routine, not
expensive in regard to materials and equipment, and
most of all, not time-consuming." One of the
challenges that the HP/DP program at Mercy Medical

Center has accepted has been to develop protocols that
require less than five minutes. "For example, you
should choose several kinds of interventions to assist
the physician to help the patient to stop smoking. It
should be something that can be done during each visit
with that patient--some self-help material that the
physician can give to the patient or some form of
counselling that he or she can do that will constantly
reinforce the change the patient is trying to make."

- Finally, in order to draw physicians to CME programs,
  the program sponsor must provide information that
  physicians can use. "You should not offer a CME
  program that emphasizes health promotion until you are
  sure that such information is relevant to the
  physicians' practices," cautions Dr. Iverson. "One of
  the easiest ways to assess this is to look at the kind
  of patients the physicians are seeing. In our
  situation," he continues, "the top ten presenting
  problems include hypertension, diabetes, smoking, and
  other life-style related conditions. About 40 percent
  of our patients are basically well patients." If 95
  percent of a physician's patients come for critical
  care, emphasizing wellness interventions "doesn't make
  sense," he concludes. Nor will a specialist be
  interested in a "wholesale" education approach; they
  will want to hear only about education strategies that
  might affect their own patients.

In addition to helping physicians develop their teaching skills, it is
important to organize the physician's immediate work environment so that it
would support and supplement that teaching. One organizational barrier that
had to be overcome before the health promotion/disease prevention program at
Mercy Medical Center (Denver, CO) could function effectively, reports Dr.
Iverson, was staff job descriptions. "In implementing health promotion
programs in our family practice clinics," he says, "we felt that all staff--not
just physicians--should play a role in teaching patients, from the receptionist
to the physician." A committee was organized to discuss this issue, and it
delineated the following teaching roles for the three individuals that
patients most often encounter during a clinic visit.

- The receptionist is responsible for giving patients a
  form in which they are encouraged to write down any
  questions they might want to ask the physician; the
  receptionist also explains any tests that the patient
  will have and also gives the patient written materials
  about those tests.

- Besides doing the normal physical examination
  procedures, the nurse reviews the questions that a
  patient has written on the question form to make sure
  the questions are clear and that they indeed ask what
  the patient wants to know. The nurse also provides the

patient with health promotion information; for example,
if the patient has come to the clinic for a well child
visit, the nurse may talk about child safety
guidelines. The nurse will also provide additional
patient education if the physician feels that this is
necessary.

. The physician's responsibility for patient education in
this setting is first to explain to the patient in
understandable, clear language the nature of the
problem, the nature of the treatment, and the patient's
responsibility in the treatment. The physician must
also answer all the questions that the patient has
written on the question form or may add during the
course of the visit. In addition, if the patient
specifically asks for advice about such a problem as
smoking, the physician follows the smoking protocol
that has been developed by the HP/DP program and helps
the patient to choose the best approach to the problem.

As Dr. Iverson points out, lack of time is a major reason why many physicians
do not include a greater teaching component in their patient care regimens.
And many of them would be glad to have someone else in their office do the
teaching, if only they were properly trained to do so. At St. Mary's Hospital
(Decatur, IL), the nursing development office, which is also responsible for
patient education activities, has developed a series of inservice training
courses that are also open to nurses who work in physicians' private offices.
During each of these sessions, the nurses can update their information on a
particular health problem, learn the teaching techniques that are used for
those patients in the hospital, and gather appropriate materials for doing the
teaching in the office setting. Physicians pay the tuition costs for their
nurse-employees, unless they themselves participate on the program faculty, in
which case their staffs' tuition is waived. Enthusiasm for the series has
been high for several obvious reasons. A less obvious benefit which had not
been anticipated is the closer communication between the office nurses and the
hospital-based nurses, who have attended the sessions together. This has
certainly enhanced continuity of care and of patient teaching as patients have
moved between the two settings.

In general, the more physicians see patient teaching materials and activities
going on around them--throughout the institution and being used by their
colleagues in the community--the more likely they are to begin integrating
these into their own patient care routine. It is therefore important to make
patient education services not only highly credible, but also highly visible.
At the University of Texas M.D. Anderson Hospital and Tumor Institute
(Houston, TX), the director of patient education responded to the medical
staff's lack of knowledge about teaching resources (self-reported in a survey
conducted by the department) by developing a mechanism to collect, review,
catalog, and display materials at several central locations in the hospital.
One area is dedicated to a pediatric learning center, another is a more
general clearinghouse for materials, and a third is a health information
center within the hospital's patient/family library. The latter collection

includes some 300 health related books. Because M.D. Anderson is a teaching institution, the education department has the opportunity to influence the patient teaching habits of new as well as more experienced physicians. The resource centers have been very useful in this regard. As their term at the hospital is completed and they prepare for independent practice, these physicians frequently stop at the centers to ask for copies of materials they have seen used at the hospital. A continuing increase in such requests has clearly reflected these physicians' growing awareness and use of available teaching tools.

Involving Physicians in Teaching in the Hospital

As physicians become more skilled in organizing the content of their messages to patients and especially as they see the beneficial effects of positive behavior change among their patients, they will tend to apply their skills more consistently. Educators can encourage this change in several ways.

- At Grady Memorial Hospital (Atlanta, GA), the patient and family education program for diabetes depends on a multidisciplinary effort that includes the physician in the teaching effort. Through notations in a patient's chart, each team member--physician, nurse, and dietitian--records the content of the teaching that went on during the most recent encounter with a patient. The team member who sees the patient next is therefore reminded to follow-up on the previous visit and to reinforce the message. One possible drawback to having three health professionals teaching the patient is the possibility that the patient may become confused by what he or she may perceive as conflicting advice. At Grady Memorial Hospital, this danger is avoided, especially in regard to diet instructions, by all the team members using a Diabetes Guidebook, which ensures that the team's teaching is coordinated and consistent.

- Physicians who don't have a great deal of confidence in their own teaching abilities may still support the concepts of patient education. Occasionally, as has happened at M.D. Anderson Hospital (Houston, TX), such physicians are willing to serve as as medical advisers to education committees and task forces. In working with these groups, some physicians have had their interest sparked in doing more teaching because they come to learn the principles by which behavior can be changed and the methods for organizing and delivering a teaching program to an individual patient or group.

- Educators who are developing inhospital group classes for specific patient populations should certainly try to include members of the medical staff on the faculty. At St. Joseph Mercy Hospital, a 60-bed institution in Centerville, IA, the physicians who have endorsed patient education and served as lecturers in prenatal, COPE, and other group teaching events have found that their interaction with patients has been enhanced by the events. Outside of the one-to-one patient/physician encounter, patients are often more willing to ask questions of physician-lecturers; some of these questions may give physicians a better idea of the information patients often need but feel constrained to ask. Furthermore, physicians who have tried the role of lecturer and enjoyed it may in turn suggest to their less interested colleagues that they do the same; so the health educator should not quickly eliminate a physician from a potential speakers' list after only one rejection.

- Another vehicle for getting physicians involved in a hospital-wide teaching effort is closed circuit television. A hospital that has even a minimum of inhouse production capabilities can put its medical staff and other professionals on the screen to deliver any one of a number of messages to its patient population. For example, the parenting education program at St. Elizabeth Hospital (Youngstown, OH) developed the script and made its own film of a Caesarean birth, in which members of the medical staff played an important role. A wider audience is planned for a series of CCTV productions at the General Ventura County Hospital (Ventura, CA). Both to inform patients about the services various departments provide and to involve members of these departments in greater CCTV use for their patients, the department of patient education is mounting a series of education/promotion "spots." Department chairmen/directors and their staffs will be the "stars" and the patient education effort should reap the benefits. At Baptist Memorial Hospital (Memphis, TN), it was a physician who decided that CCTV would be a useful tool to teach nurses how to do preoperative teaching with open heart patients. This physician, who does the most by-pass surgery in the hospital, noticed inconsistencies in the information nurses were communicating. With the help of the CCTV staff, the physician arranged "screen tests," during which each nurse conducted a teaching session with a real patient. The nurse who demonstrated the best approach "won" the test, and her film was then used to teach others. The physician also convinced other cardiovascular surgeons and the patient education committee to use the film for patient teaching via CCTV. The success of this venture has impressed some other members of the medical staff, several of whom have approached the patient education department with similar plans.

Involving Physicians in Communitywide Teaching

The positive exposure that physicians may get in the process of lecturing or otherwise talking to community groups is probably the best incentive for physicians' becoming involved in communitywide teaching. Some physicians may already know how to create such opportunities for themselves. Others may be eager to do so, especially if they consider such appearances to be good marketing in a competitive medical practice environment. Again, hospital-based educators, especially if they are well connected within a network of community agencies, can be a great help in linking interested groups with willing physicians.

- A common technique, especially in smaller communities where the hospital is the only major health-related institution, is a speakers' bureau. In fact, doing a survey of the medical staff members to gather information on each one's favorite lecture topic is also a good basis for developing information about potential committee members for hospital-based education activities. If the education department is given some responsibility for allocating speaking slots or otherwise choosing a physician to fill an invitation, the choice must be a scrupulously fair but also an appropriate one. Too many failures at this matchmaking can render a speakers' bureau inactive, and an educator new to a community and to a medical staff may do well to seek the advice of others in the hospital (the community relations department, for example) before confirming any plans.

- Just as physicians often need help in developing their one-to-one patient education skills, some of them can also use some advice on sharpening their techniques for making group presentations. Pat Herje, director of health education at Jackson Clinic, a group practice in Madison, WI, spends quite a bit of time working with physicians on their presentations to community groups.[4] Visual material in the form of slides and printed matter are always a large part of each presentation, and Herje keeps physicians to a strict schedule for developing these to meet printing and other processing deadlines for program brochures and hand-outs. She also helps them practice their presentations, often in front of a group of other clinic staff members or on a video tape, so that the presentation can then be evaluated and practical

suggestions made for improvement. Most physicians who
go through this proces the first time dislike it very
much, Herje reports; but they soon realize how much
more effective they become as speakers and they come to
appreciate her skills and her role as organizer and
coordinator of the clinic's programs in community
education. Her efforts have also helped physicians to
communicate better with local media; a workshop Herje
organized for physicians gave them the opportunity to
discuss with representatives of local newspapers,
radio, and television the kinds of information they are
most often interested in finding. Tapes of samples
interviews between physicians and media representatives
were also shown and gave all the participants the
opportunity to discuss their perceptions of the quality
and process of local reporting of medical/health care
issues.

. Communities with cable networks, with public radio and
television stations, and generally with other mass
media outlets for health-related information are full
of opportunities for the health educator to encourage
physician involvement in community health education.
For example, if a physician has been involved in
developing a closed circuit television program
appropriate for a general audience, it could be offered
to a local cable network for its public service
programming. Again, the educator could enlist the help
of the hospital's public relations staff to search out
the best medium and then to arrange for a physician to
appear in it.

Obviously, a educator's willingness to use any of these approaches will depend
a great deal both on time available and on the degree to which the current
level of health promotion activities matches the department's goals. It may
appear that a smoothly running department with a reasonably comprehensive set
of programs and good physician support does not need to involve physicians in
any more teaching. The idea may seem superfluous; in some institutions, it
may even be--mistakenly--considered disruptive. But it is an idea that
educators should seriously consider, because many newly trained physicians are
already considering it on their own. A hospital in which a system is already
being developed to foster cooperation between physicians and other patient
teachers will be best prepared to offer an integrated approach to health
promotion.

References

1. Adamson, T., and others. A community program to link physicians and
    patient education. PROCAP-Professional Competence Assurance Program for
    Practicing Physicians. San Francisco, CA: University of California
    School of Medicine, 1982.

2. PROCAP.

3. Iverson, D. Personal communication, April 29, 1983.

4. Herje, P. Personal communication, June 27, 1983.

Chapter 9

WORKING WITH PHYSICIANS: HOW TO BEGIN

As the early portions of this book clearly define it, our goal has been to help hospital-based educators to work with physicians in developing and delivering effective health promotion programs. By describing their experiences to us, both educators and physicians have helped us to achieve much of this goal--to provide others in the field with examples of how physician involvement has been successfully encouraged and effectively organized. Their combined and cumulative experience has also served to strengthen an early hypothesis into a conviction--which is that, in seeking physicians' support of health promotion programs, the question is not whether one should do it, but how.

In fact, the notion that more productive interaction is needed among physicians, other health care professionals, and other hospital decision makers is becoming incorporated into the popular wisdom of many of these groups. Physicians are joining hospital administrators at seminars that urge both groups to cooperate more than ever in ensuring their institutions' competitive position in their communities.[1] Leaders in the medical profession, appreciating the importance of physicians' understanding of hospital operations and of hospital administrators' understanding of medical staff concerns, propose to facilitate that understanding by recommending that all hospital administrative committees have physician members and all medical staff committees include members from hospital administration.[2] If it is successful, this effort should have a direct impact on the degree to which physicians participate in all hospital programming, health promotion included. Some coordinators of community education and wellness programs already report that their administrators and/or governing boards are pointedly suggesting that physician input be invited for programs that have been successful without it. Their primary objective in making these suggestions is to draw physicians more into the organizational life of the institution, to make its goals become as much as possible their goals, so that hospitals and all who work in them can respond in a coordinated and effective way to the pressures of health care delivery.

With this trend in mind, it seems possible to predict that all health promotion programs, whether they currently seem to need it or not, will eventually benefit to a greater or lesser degree from physician participation. If the advantages of nurturing physician support are not immediately felt by one program, they will more than likely be enjoyed in a later effort. The point is, a beginning must be made. Analysis of a specific program's needs may suggest that physician involvement in planning is not crucial. Assessment of a potential population for another program may indicate that physician referral will not constitute a major source of program users. However, a thorough study of the current effectiveness and future needs of the health promotion department and of the institution will invariably reveal the wisdom of cooperating with physicians, who will continue to be major providers of care and major decision-makers in the way it is provided by others.

This book describes many ways in which others have organized physician support of health promotion programming—many more ways than any one program coordinator would wish to apply and many more than would be appropriate for any one program or institution. However, a few of the guidelines that grow out of others' successful experiences are so basic as to be considered generic: they can be applied with good results to every kind of health promotion program, whether it be patient education, employee health, or community health and wellness programs.

The first of these, as Chapter 5 describes, is to find at least one physician advocate who can serve as liaison between the medical staff and the hospitalwide health promotion effort. The kind of relationship that will be most appropriate will depend on a variety of factors, many of which are described in earlier parts of this book. For example, if a medical staff is very interested in a program for a particular patient group, the best approach may be to establish a formal relationship with one of the physician as medical advisor for that program. Such an arrangement may give the physicians the degree of control they want over program content and delivery, while it provides program staff the opportunity to consistently communicate with the medical staff and to establish confidence and trust. On the other hand, if physicians are for the most part neutral about a program and the program itself does not seem to be suffering from lack of their input, it is nonetheless wise to investigate the possibilities that cooperation with physicians may offer an advisory position to the program or an advisory group may provide the mechanism for doing so.

This same mechanism may provide the form for physician input into program review, planning, and development of materials. Organizing such input—to discover their interests and needs—is a second essential step in a health promotion staff's working with physicians. Again, it is not so much the form of their input but the fact of it that is important. Many educators have found surveys of physicians' attitudes and needs to be an excellent beginning to defining the programs that physicians are most likely to support and in the development of which they are most likely to join.

A sense of how physicians may respond to various aspects of a health promotion department's activities will also help the staff to take a third important step in developing a good working relationship with the medical staff; that is, to discover if there are any issues of such concern to physicians that they must be dealt with immediately. For example, if physicians are generally suspicious about a department's abilities to develop useful programs, the source of this suspicion must be discovered and eliminated. It may stem from a program that was poorly developed by a previous patient education coordinator, or it may be the previous coordinator's lack of tact in dealing with some physicians on the medical staff. Whatever breach has been created in the relationship between the medical staff and the health promotion staff must be healed before they can work together closely and well. The healing will seldom occur spontaneously: it must be thoughtfully planned and patiently applied if it is to change the habits and attitudes that have been taken considerably long periods to develop.

Opportunities Offered by External Incentives

While patience is required in this process, the ability to capture the moment is also very useful. Recognizing an unusual opportunity to serve physicans' needs while also accomplishing a department's goals may help to win some new allies among the medical staff who previously saw little value in the relationship. This point is well demonstrated by the example of the physicians who began to see the need for community health education when a chiropractor started to offer health classes for consumers (see Chapter 6). The educator at the community hospital was able to offer her services to the physicians by organizing opportunities for them to provide correct health-related information to community residents. In the process, the physicians came to better understand the community's constant need for such information and to support the hospital's efforts to provide it. A similar opportunity may arise if a physician group is planning to form or join a preferred provider organization; especially if they and the hospital will be joining efforts in such a venture, the educator has the opportunity to demonstrate to the physicians how incorporating patient education into their practice can make the physician group more attractive providers to potential business and industrial clients.

Discovering and using such incentives to pique physicians' interest and to engage their participation demands the kind of knowledge of the medical staff, the institution, and the environment that is described in the first four chapters of this book. Productive action cannot be taken until at least some of this knowledge is accumulated.

A Final Word

It would be impossible to outline in a document such as we have produced here exactly the steps that a particular health promotion staff must take if they discover that their medical staff and their institution demonstrate characteristics "w, x, and y" but not "z." Beyond our offering recommendations that can be useful in the early phases of seeking physician support, more specific prescribing must be left to the participants themselves. Perhaps only one more piece of advice can be given--and it probably cannot be emphasized enough: much of the success of the formula that educators will choose to apply in their institutions will depend on their own attitude toward the physicians whose support they seek. If the reason they approach physicians is to use them, then they will most probably be less effective than the educators who anticipate and offer mutual benefits from cooperation with the medical staff. There is of course much to be said for developing a practical sense for what will work and what will not, despite all generous efforts at understanding and compromise. Such occasional losses notwithstanding, the educator who extends the hand of cooperation and seeks support in reaching a commonly held goal will find that knowledgeable, reasonable physicians will be ready to respond.

References

1. Lefton, D. Hospital administration seek medical staff cooperation. *American Medical News*. March 18, 1983.

2. Resolution: 50 (A-83), American Medical Association, House of Delegates, 1983.

PART III

CASE STUDIES

CASE STUDY 1

INCORPORATING PATIENT EDUCATION INTO PHYSICIANS'
QUALITY ASSURANCE ACTIVITIES

In the broadest sense, the assurance of high quality in health care demands
that two results be achieved in the encounter between a provider and a
client. One is that medical knowledge be applied properly and without
error.[1] The other is that the patient be satisfied with what has taken
place, a perception that involves "what patients and providers expect of each
other, what happens between the patient and the provider, how the patient
understands and reacts to what takes place," and "what role the environment
plays in this interaction.[2]

Physicians learn through training and experience how to be thorough in the
technical interventions they choose to apply both in diagnosis and
treatment--how to apply medical knowledge properly and without error. To
assess the quality of these interventions in a particular hospital, many
medical staffs have developed formal quality assurance mechanisms (QA); some
of these mechanisms also include components that are designed to bring about
improvement in the performance of physicians whose work falls below
institutional QA standards.[3] Just as physicians have not consistently
included patient education in their patient care regimens, so also is it true
that physicians have rarely included patient education criteria in their
standards for judging quality of care. For example, in a study of one kind of
activity that is often included in quality assurance--the medical audit,
researchers discovered that only four percent of 6,662 medical audit criteria
that had been applied to 448 audit procedures were related to patient
education.[4] Another three percent were related to other psychosocial
aspects of care--psychosocial history, psychosocial consultation, and impact
of illness. The remaining 93 percent of the criteria were related to the
technical aspects of diagnosis and treatment.

The authors of the medical audit research suggest that the QA mechanism can be
a valuable tool for incorporating patient education into the comprehensive
treatment of illness. In particular, they speculate that some areas may
benefit more than others by inclusion of patient education and other
psychosocial interventions; these areas include "health maintenance,
life-threatening or chronic illness, psychiatric illness, illness that demands
a change in a life-style and instances where there is evidence of psychosocial
or social breakdown in the patient or family.

Paul B. Batalden, M.D., whose research in the area has led him to co-author a
book of specific guidelines on implementing quality assurance in ambulatory
care settings, reports that, in his experience with his own institution as
well as others, "the quality assurance mechanism has been a driving force in
getting a broader commitment to health education."[5] This has been the case
because the performance that the QA mechanism is designed to evaluate consists
of the combined behavior of the physician, the patient, and the support staff;
therefore, the goal of the QA program "is to induce and secure favorable
changes in the behavior of all three."[6] Patient education must therefore be
an integral part of the process.

Problem seeking. The QA process in any institution generally begins by the search for a problem in the way care has been delivered. At St. Louis Park Medical Center (Minneapolis, MN), where Dr. Batalden is program director for the Health Services Research Center, several different mechanisms are used in this first phase, in addition to the most frequently used tool of medical chart review. One of these mechanisms is telephone interviews of patients, conducted by a registered nurse; Dr. Batalden reports that the medical center's quality assurance effort has by this point developed approximately 50 different telephone interview protocols. "If you ask patients, as part of the QA enterprise, about the quality of care that they receive," he says, "then you open up an enormous avenue of direct feedback about the adequacy of the patient's understanding about the condition, or the medications, or the other parts of treatment." For example, the telephone interview process was used to evaluate the care of allergy patients; their responses indicated that they were all more or less uncertain about the medications they were to take--their purpose, side-effects, and so on. This discovery led specifically to the development of a patient education handout that would reinforce the information patients were given during their visit. As this example suggests, Dr. Batalden continues, "learning from the consumer's perspective about the health care that they have received and the kind of care that they would like to have received has been a seedbed for literally dozens of health education efforts."

Problem formulation. A problem is not always so easily defined as the previous example suggests. At St. Louis Park Medical Center, for instance, the high utilization of the center's pediatric services for such conditions as upper respiratory infections (URI) seemed to stem from confusion about how care should be given at home. "The impetus to find out why patients were not using services appropriately came from the doctors themselves," reports Dr. Batalden. A QA staff person was assigned to discover what were the sources of patient's information about self-care; she used a structured interview technique to ask each pediatrician and pediatric nurse the kind of instructions that they gave to patients and parents of patients with URI. The multiplicity of viewpoints that was discovered through this process was clearly the reason for the confusion and for the inappropriate use of the center's services.

Problem resolution. To arrive at one set of instructions that could be consistently given in all cases of URI, Dr. Batalden reports, the pediatric department went through a modified nominal group technique until they arrived at a consensus of how best to instruct a patient to manage the condition and so to make wiser use of health services.

Such cooperation in arriving at a solution differentiates a QA process that involves everyone in change from a process that merely dictates it. Unlike a QA method that requires only a committee or a small segment of the medical staff to do the work, the QA process at the St. Louis Park Medical Center enables all the physicians to participate in problem definition and resolution. The fact that almost 100 percent of them do participate has a direct bearing on the center's incorporation of patient education into treatment protocols.

"We involve physicians in the development of education materials," says Dr. Batalden, "so they don't feel as if somebody from Mars is telling them what to teach patients. The education staff serves as resource developers, whose role is to listen to many different points of view and to reflect those with the appropriate words in the appropriate form."

Working with the QA Committee

At East Tennessee Children's Hospital (Knoxville, TN), reports Laura Borden, R.N., Child Life Coordinator, the Medical Quality Assurance Committee asks each patient care department to cooperate in the QA process by presenting the committee with a list of relevant problems that it has identified for study.[7] Such a list is developed at the beginning of every year; the committee then reviews each list, prioritizes the topics, and gives each department a schedule for making presentations about those topics to the committee during its monthly conferences. The committee is chaired by the chief-elect of the medical staff; the assistant administrator for patient care also serves on the committee, along with 20 physicians (among them, the chiefs of surgery and of medicine, who are also medical advisors to the patient education function).

The annual topics list from patient education is developed with a variety of inputs, Ms. Borden says, and not least of these is experience with what the department has accomplished so far and knowledge of its goals and objectives. Informal communication with the medical and nursing staff is another source of information about needs that the education department can fill. For example, by talking with physicians, Ms. Borden discovered that parents of children who were being sent home with apnea monitors were not receiving consistent instructions. To get a better idea of the degree to which this was a problem, Ms. Borden asked the medical records department to audit appropriate charts. The results led her to add this issue to the list she presented for the QA committee's consideration.

Normally, her list of topics brings her to a QA conference three or four times a year, Ms. Borden says, although the committee is very receptive to requests for an invitation at other times, if a pressing matter arises. To prepare for a presentation, Ms. Borden gathers statistics about the problem (such as those from an audit), relevant literature and descriptions about the experience of other hospitals, a proposal for resolving the problem (such as a policy that standardizes instructions about apnea monitors and infant CPR), and possibly teaching materials that could be used to implement the policy. As was the case with the apnea monitor issue, the committee may ask her either to bring more information to the next meeting, or to revise the proposed solution, or perhaps to develop other teaching materials. The process has worked well, Ms. Borden concludes, and it has made a considerable difference in how aware physicians are about the information needs of their patients.

Most quality assurance activities in hospitals have not reached the sophistication that Dr. Bataldem describes, nor are they as willing to accept the input of educators, as Ms. Borden reports. If the QA process in an institution is conducted in the now more traditional way-by a medical audit committee, the issue of patient education can still be injected into the proceedings. If the education staff is not invited to participate, the department's medical advisor could make recommendations to the committee about developing appropriate criteria for including patient education in the treatment of specific conditions. "There are all kinds of 'tracer' conditions that point to the failure of patient education," says John Renner, M.D., director of St. Mary Family Medicine Center, Kansas City, MO. "Let's just take the readmission rate for someone who's had a coronary who continues to smoke. If you don't set up an option for that patient to help him stop smoking, you have done that patient irreparable harm." In developing criteria for evaluating the care of such patients, then, someone on the QA committee--be it a physician or a nurse or an educator--must constantly ask and have formalized patient education questions. However, "if the QA mechanism in a hospital is limited to counting incidents in medical records, it's useless," he says. "There's little to be learned there either for quality assurance purposes or for patient education, and the health educator is wasting time by pursuing that route." It may be more productive to first establish a link with some marketing function, Dr. Bataldem says, with some department that is listening to what patients are saying about what they need. "Use whatever mechanism the institution has for getting at patients' perceptions--use market research studies, use long-range planning feedback, use the satisfaction-with-care surveys. Whatever the institution calls quality assurance may not be what is really done in quality assurance," Dr. Bataldem concludes, "so educators must think more broadly about the term to mean improving quality of care through feedback from patients and doctors and staff."

One example of a different kind of quality assurance comes from Baptist Hospital of Miami, where no intervention on the part of the patient education staff was necessary to convince emergency department physicians and nursing staff that discharge instructions were an important part of the medical record.[9] Although giving ED patients discharge instructions was standard practice, in at least one case, a copy of the instructions did not appear in the medical record. The hospital became concerned when a patient alleged that she had not been given discharge instructions and claimed to have suffered some injury as a result. Therefore, the ED head nurse and the ED physicians expanded the number of preprinted discharge instructions. In addition, the policy was reinforced that patients and family sign that they have received and understand the instructions. The instructions with the patient's signature are retained in the medical record as well as given to the patient.

In the above example, the patient's expression of a need for information emphasizes Dr. Bataldem's point that feedback from patients is a powerful spur for accelerating patient education efforts as well as generally improving provider-patient communication. As Chapter 1 suggests, patient satisfaction depends as much on a patient's perception of the quality of care as on the measurable competence with which that care was rendered. Baptist Hospital of Miami provides another example of how patient education can fill first the needs of a particular patient group but also ensure the hospital against potential risk.

According to Leah Kinnaird, R.N., director of the hospital's patient and community education department, "one instance in which we applied risk management principles before there was any litigation was in developing a bereavement support team." The team, which consists of obstetrical nurses, childbirth educators, a physician, and a chaplain, organizes and facilitates the discussions of a support group for parents whose newborns have died. Although the medical staff approved the development of this team, Ms. Kinnaird recalls, some physicians were skeptical about its value and did not want their patients to participate. It occurred to her that physicians might be concerned that something a team member might say during a group session might jeopardize either a physician or the hospital. The hospital's risk management consultant, Patricia Blanco, R.N., was asked to present a program to team members, outlining the role of patient education in hospital risk management. The team members were able to see how the special attention which they give to patients in a time of grief has a secondary gain of decreasing the physician's and hospital's risk exposure. Since Kinnaird reported to the physicians that the team had met with the risk management consultant, both physicians and hospital staff have seen the value of the bereavement team and physicians now uniformly refer their patients to the service.

Education for Assuring Quality Care

Once a problem is identified, both the risk management and the quality assurance mechanisms should include a method to help providers improve either their own performance or the performance of the system by which care is delivered. Sometimes, the change may require only a single intervention, such as establishing a policy that patients sign a form after they have given appropriate discharge instructions. In other instances, the performance to be modified may be of longer standing and may require a continuing effort, and it may be that the effort entails some kind of education for physicians.

At St. Vincent's Hospital in Portland, OR, Barbara Main, director of educational services, did not use a formal quality assurance mechanism to identify a deficit in the medical staff's knowledge of the department's programs.[10] However, her frequent contact with physicians as the staff member who provides support to the continuing medical education committee led her to conclude that physicians needed to be better informed--not only about the fact that programs were available, but about their quality. Because grand rounds are a traditional medium for physicians to receive this kind of information, she decided to use it to describe some specific programs.

Main asked the head of the department of medicine to add two sessions on these programs to the grand rounds schedule, which is normally planned several months in advance. At St. Vincent's Hospital, Main reports, the waiting period is often as long as six months. She and several of her staff attended a few grand rounds conferences "to find out what the right tone and techniques" were in their institution. They found that the lecture form with slides was used most frequently, and they adopted this form for their own presentations. One of the two sessions was devoted to describing the smoking cessation program at St. Vincent's Hospital. Main provided statistics on program results among previous participants, compared the methodology used in the program to other techniques, and supported her statements with liberal references from the medical literature. It is more effective to quote from medical literature than from patient education literature when addressing physicians, Main emphasizes. The education staff also assembled packets of literature about all the department's programs, and these were distributed to the approximately 50 physicians who attended, out of a total of about 200 potential participants. Receiving continuing medical education credits was doubtless an attractive feature of the program, Main speculates, but being assured of a credible program is also important when physicians are deciding whether a program is worth attending.

Such credibility can be assured by involving physicians in planning programs for physicians. When Anne Stechmann, M.A., coordinator for patient education for the Veterans' Administration North Central Regional Medical Center (Minneapolis, MN), identified a need to provide administrative-level physicians with information related to increasing physician involvement in patient education, she relied on physicians at the center as well as physician-liaisons in V.A. medical centers to help plan the most appropriate educational approaches for meeting the objective. These physicians identified particular topics that would be important to include in the conference (for example, physician's legal responsibility) and selected several physicians with a national reputation to make presentations. The planning committee was clearly identified on the brochure that invited registration to the two-day conference. The degree of physician involvement in planning and presenting the conference was significant in attracting participants and in giving the conference credibility, says Stechmann.[11]

Arranging CME Credit. As in the example from St. Vincent's Hospital, another source of attraction for the V.A. program was its granting of CME credit toward a Physician's Recognition Award of the American Medical Association. The right to extend such credit is granted by state medical societies, schools of medicine, and other organizations that have been accredited by the Accreditation Council for Continuing Medical Education (ACCME).[12] An institution such as a hospital may already have ACCME accreditation to sponsor programs that grant CME credit. If not, an educator who is interested in planning such a program can find out information about sponsorship requirements and other relevant matters from the state medical society or one of its local chapters.

A hospital's association with a residency program offers several advantages in providing continuing medical education. In addition to being affiliated with an accredited sponsor of CME programs, the hospital has easier access to guest lecturers who visit the medical school to speak to students. These lecturers may be a major attraction to a physician audience as well, so a health educator in such a hospital should follow guest lecture schedules and use them when it may be appropriate. In particular, if a program is being offered to residents, it may also attract attending physicians who wish to have access to the most current information. This is a useful strategy for another important reason, points out Donald Iverson, Ph.D., director of the health promotion/ disease prevention program at Mercy Medical Center, Denver, CO.[13] "If you are trying to influence one group of practitioners in a hospital (in this case, the residents)," he explains, "then it is also important to promote the same kind of practice among others (attending physicians, for example), so that the program's influence on the residents is not neutralized every time they work alongside attending physicians who are either unfamiliar or unsupportive of the principles of health promotion."

In this way, the assurance of high quality care can come full circle--from problem identification through the formulation of solutions to the ongoing improvement of performance, which may sometimes be achieved through continuing education for the medical staff. And the educator, by using the mechanisms for change that both the institution and the medical staff have legitimized, can help physicians to better understand and accept the principles and practice of health promotion.

References

1. Batalden, P. and O'Connor, J. Quality Assurance in Ambulatory Care. Germantown, MD: Aspen Systems Corporation, 1980.

2. Quality Assurance.

3. Baker, F. Quality assurance and program evaluation. Evaluation and the Health Professions. 6:149-160, June 1983.

4. Berg, J. and Kelly, J. Evaluation of psychosocial health care in quality assurance. Medical Care. 19:24-29, Jan. 1981.

5. Batalden, P., M.D. Personal communication, June 2, 1983.

6. Quality Assurance.

7. Borden, L. Personal communication, January 14 and June 13, 1983.

8. Renner, J., M.D. Personal communication, May 17, 1983.

9. Kinnaird, L., R.N. Personal communication, May 19, 1983.

10. Main, B. Personal communication, June 27, 1983.

11. Stechmann, A. Personal communication, June 10, 1983.

12. American Medical Association. The Physician's Recognition Award, Information Booklet 1983. Chicago: The AMA, 1983.

13. Iverson, D., Ph.D. Personal communication, April 29, 1983.

CASE STUDY 2

USING SURVEYS TO GENERATE PHYSICIAN SUPPORT

Finding out what physicians think about health promotion and what kind of
health promotion programs they think their community needs serves two
important functions. First, the results of such a needs assessment process
can help to identify and shape programs that physicians are likely to
recommend to their patients. Second, the process itself can generate many
opportunities for increased communication with physicians, for their growing
more familiar with and confident in educators' capabilities, and consequently
for drawing physicians into the planning and delivery of health promotion
programs. The process of gathering information from physicians can be as
simple and informal or as sophisticated and formal as the situation requires
and as resources permit.

The Simple Survey

Educators who first take on the responsibilities of program coordinator often
find that a simple survey instrument, in the form of a written questionnaire
administered to physicians, is a very useful indicator of their interests and
needs. When Dena Baskin became patient education coordinator at Day Kimball
Hospital (Putnam, CT), there were no organized, standardized education
services for patients.[1] To give her work a relevant direction, Baskin
decided to ask physicians and nurses on the hospital's staff what they thought
would be the most useful educational programs to begin providing to patients.
The physicians were given a list of some of the more traditional and widely
used programs (such as diabetes education, cardiac rehabilitation, and the
like) and were asked to check those that would (a) most benefit their patients
and (b) most likely increase compliance with prescribed courses of treatment.
The questionnaire to nurses was more open-ended (i.e., they were asked to list
useful program topics rather than to check them off a list already provided).
A comparison of the two sets of results clearly showed an overlap in the needs
that the two groups perceived among their patients. The weight of their
opinions, as well as the fact that successful delivery of a new education
program would depend on close cooperation with physicians and nurses, led
Baskin to choose a diabetic teaching program as her first priority.

The survey results were also useful in another regard, Baskin reports,
"because they helped to identify the physicians who would be likely supporters
of a diabetic teaching program." As she began to develop program materials,
Baskin "filtered them through those physicians who had expressed an interest
in such a program." In this way, she began to forge some early links in a
communications network with the hospital's medical staff. When she later
wanted some physician input regarding a possible outpatient diabetic teaching
program, her earlier survey results helped her to reach those physicians in
whose practice such a program would be most relevant.

A survey of this kind is "simple" in several ways.

- It is short, so that physicians are not apt to put it
  aside because they are too busy.

- It does not require interpretation on the physician's part, so it is easy to fill out.

- The results do not lend themselves to easy misinterpretation, so they can be used as guides in programming with reasonable assurance that they really do represent physicians' interests and intentions.

- No sophisticated knowledge of survey instruments is essential here; a simple counting of which program topics are checked most often is a good indicator.

- Finally, the matching of results from this survey with those from the nursing staff helps avoid the possibility that a new program will become a point of disagreement between two important groups of providers of care.

Some More Extensive Instruments

A longer, more open-ended questionnaire may take some more time to construct and analyze, but it can provide more information for program planning. When Margaret Bazeley became the patient health education coordinator at the Veterans Administration Medical Center in Saginaw, MI, she found herself in a position similar to the one Baskin describes.[2] Attempting an informal survey of needs through individual meetings with physicians and chiefs of service (department heads), Bazeley sensed that "no one had a good overall perception of needs. What was needed to get patient education activities organized on an institution-wide basis was a good baseline," she reports, so that the needs that surfaced could be prioritized. Because she was also looking for a vehicle to demonstrate those needs to others with whom she would have to work--such as the physicians and the multidisciplinary patient education advisory committee--she decided to administer three different questionnaires: one to physicians, another to patients, and a third to non-physician staff who were involved in patient education activities.

The 13 questions on the physician questionnaire (see page 85), were designed to elicit several different kinds of information. As Bazeley writes in her report on the survey findings, the questionnaire asked physicians to report on their level of input and referral of patients to education programs and on their awareness of existing patient education programs; it also asked for suggestions for new offerings. Portions of it dealt with the benefits to the patients from attending classes and the reasons that physicians perceived for patients not benefitting from classes.

To help assure that the questionnaire would elicit the kind of information she intended, Bazeley submitted it for review to a "jury" of eight individuals-- among them, other coordinators, a chief of nursing service, and a chief of dental service. After making the minor corrections the jury had suggested, Bazeley field tested the questionnaire by administering it in person to three physicians on the staff of the medical center; one worked with inpatients, another with outpatients, and a third was a chief of a service "who had a handle on administrative considerations."

Although the field testing did not lead to any major change in the questionnaire (she did change the sequence of a few questions to permit a more logical flow in the information), Bazeley reports discovering that her initial intention to personally administer the questionnaire proved too cumbersome. Despite the fact that she had appointments for completing the questionnaire with each of the three physicians, she was often "bumped" from the schedule by the physicians' having to see patients. Although the medical staff at the institution consists of only 24 full-time physicians, Bazeley decided to mail the questionnaire through the intra-institutional mail and ask physicians to complete it themselves. This approach eliminated the need for a great deal of time for administering the survey in person.

The response rate--83%--was a good one, and Bazeley attributes this to the fact that she spent some time preparing physicians for the forthcoming survey. She asked the chief of staff to put her on the agenda of a monthly medical staff meeting, where she described the purpose of the survey and speculated how the results might be helpful in improving patient education services.

The report of survey findings is a lengthy, detailed document that contains not only descriptions of the questionnaire design, the questionnaires themselves, and an interpretation of the results. This report was distributed to the patient education advisory committee (which includes one physician) as well as to the chief of medical services, the chief of surgery, the chief of staff of the medical center, and the medical center director. On the basis of the findings, Bazeley drafted a formal plan of action for the following year; this document lists ten recommendations in order of priority, delineates specific objectives related to each, identifies necessary resources to accomplish them, and sets deadlines.

The two documents--the survey report and the action plan--have been very useful in generating a good deal of support, and much of this has come from the medical staff. Before the survey process was begun, Bazeley says, most staff physicians were not aware of the variety of decentralized education programs that were in place. Yet, as the survey demonstrated, they felt a great deal of frustration with patients who were not complying with treatment regimens and who were consequently becoming "chronic repeaters." The survey helped Bazeley to become known as the patient education coordinator, to develop linkages for consistent communication with physicians and others, and to foster a new interest and willingness among physicians to serve as consultants to subcommittees that will be implementing the objectives described in the action plan. A related occurrence that has indirectly increased physicians' confidence in the benefits of patient education programming has been the increased activity in the various services or departments that normally deliver the programs to patients. The survey process and the report of results generated a great deal of discussion about patient education, says Bazeley, and various departments have taken it upon themselves to make changes that would facilitate the delivery or improve the content of patient education programs.

Finding Help in Developing Surveys

As the survey sample gets larger and as the possibilities for bias and other kinds of misinterpretation increase, it becomes more important to apply the rules of instrument development to help avoid such skewing of survey results. For example, when one is trying to discover relationships among responses (such as the relationship between physicians' specialty and their positive attitudes toward certain health promotion programs), a more complex analysis is required than one would use in simply counting the number of times physicians expressed interest in a specific program. In particular when a survey is being developed for evaluation or other kinds of formal research, instrument construction requires skills that most educators in health promotion have not acquired.

It is possible to identify when such skills are necessary by referring to some publications in the field; Locating Resources for Evaluation is one guide to many of these.[3] It is also possible to acquire such skills through association with experts who have them. For example, as a chapter in this book reports, the cardiac rehabilitation program at Baptist Memorial Hospital (Memphis, TN) was developed in part on the basis of a survey of physicians in the community. The survey was conducted by a research firm retained for that purpose; in addition to generating useful information for program development, the firm's involvement provided not only research capabilities to the project, but also lent the results the objectivity and credibility that made them acceptable to the physicians.

Individual consultants can also serve this purpose and may often be found on university facilities. For example, the survey of community physicians that was conducted by the Lexington County Hospital, (West Columbia, SC) was developed by the project director of the hospital's community health education grant, in consultation with a public health faculty member from the University of South Carolina. Additional input came from other hospital health education personnel, the hospital health planner, and the hospital community health education committee (which included some physician members).[4]

The potential sample for this survey consisted of all primary care physicians (a total of 72) who were serving Lexington County Hospital in an active or courtesy capacity; they represented general practice as well as the specialties of family practice, pediatrics, internal medicine, obstetrics and gynecology, and emergency medicine. The survey's first objective was to measure physician perceptions of the community's health status in terms of illness prevalence and associated lifestyle and environmental factors. Its second objective was to assess the willingness of these physicians to refer their patients to community health education lifestyle intervention programs.

The availability of expert help in survey analysis permitted the project director to draw conclusions from the survey that could be statistically supported. For example, the survey report suggests that "1) specialization in family practice or internal medicine, 2) board certification, 3) affiliation with a group practice, and/or 4) having practiced medicine for less than five years may be characteristic of current positive referral attitudes among primary care physicians at Lexington County Hospital." This information helped the project staff to anticipate and nurture the most likely sources of physician support as they planned the programs that the survey results had justified as most needed.

Ensuring a Good Response Rate

The survey that Christine Brown, R.N., conducted for the Well Being, a health promotion center associated with the Scripps Memorial Hospital Foundation (LaJolla, CA) attempted not only to find out whether physicians would be willing to refer patients to the centers programs but to encourage them to do so.[5] As the program's director, Brown wished to provide incentives to physicians to tell their patients about appropriate programs. One such incentive was to establish a reciprocal referral network, by which the center would provide to information about physicians in the community to its clients who did not have physicians; the individuals then made their own choice of physicians to consult. The information about physicians' services, office hours, insurance arrangements, and so forth was gathered from the first set of questions in the survey (see questionnaire, page 87). The fact that the questionnaire gave physicians the opportunity to enter this information into the center's referral files was an added incentive for them to return the mailed questionnaire. A letter appended to the questionnaire reminded physicians about the various aspects of the center, which had already been described to them on previous occasions. The letter emphasized the importance of the physicians' involvement in the "participative planning" of future center programs and thanked them for their help.

Other examples of survey instruments that offer direct benefit to physicians by way of encouraging their response include several that ask for information about physicians' interest in participating in a speakers' bureau. A separate questionnaire can certainly be developed to gather just this information. However, appending it to a few questions about physicians' attitudes or referral patterns can serve both a program's and physicians' interest. If some physicians are experiencing a decrease in volume of office practice or are otherwise interested in making themselves more visible in the community, the opportunity to join a hospital-sponsored speakers' bureau may be a very attractive offer.

The Personal Approach to Surveys

Leah S. Kinnaird, R.N., director of patient and community education at Baptist Hospital of Miami, Inc. (Miami, FL), assures good response rates on many surveys by collecting the responses herself.[6] "I meet with physicians all the time," she reports, and she often interviews them about new program proposals. On the basis of these interviews, she draws up reports that she presents to various physician meetings. "If I can read to the whole group the positive responses they each made individually," Kinnaird says, "they're much more likely to support me as a group."

Kinnaird used this approach to gain approval for a post-mastectomy discussion group. She interviewed 11 general surgeons who perform mastectomies and drew up a report indicating that 10 of them approved of a discussion program that would be led by a psychologist. She presented this report to a meeting of the surgery department, where none of the interviewed physicians changed their opinions. Some aspects of the program that some of them had disapproved were also discussed and modifications suggested; accepting their negative opinions as well as their positive opinions is important, Kinnaird emphasizes, not only to ensure the quality of the program but also to reassure physician that all their input is being considered in program planning.

Approaching physicians on an individual basis seems to work well with proposals that are new to physicians, Kinnaird suggests, "with ideas that they may not have thought of themselves. If reaching each one individually would be too time-consuming, then some other approach should be used," she continues. "For example, I wouldn't do a survey like this for a type of surgery that every doctor in an institution does."

As Kinnaird says, in such a case, another approach must be found. Because to work effectively with physicians, most health promotion programs demand that an educator constantly communicate with physicians, and survey questionnaires are an excellent way to begin the dialogue.

References

1. Baskin, D., R.N. Personal communication, June 21, 1983.

2. Bazeley, M. Personal communication, June 23, 1983.

3. Zapka, J., and others. Locating Resources for Evaluation. Chicago, IL: American Hospital Association, 1982. Two resources listed in this guide that may be of special interest are: Fink, A. and Kosecoff, J. How to Evaluate Education Programs: A Compilation of Ideas that Work. Washington, DC: Capitol Publications, Inc., 1980; and Moser, C. and Kalton, G. Survey Methods in Social Investigation. London: Heinemann Educational Books, 1975.

4. Mullen, K. and G. Costello. Primary care physicians as a source of health education needs assessment data. Unpublished report, Community Health Education Demonstration Project, Lexington County Hospital, West Columbia, SC, 1981.

5. Brown, C., R.N. Personal communication, March 25, 1983.

6. Kinnaird, L., R.N. Personal communication, May 19, 1983.

Veterans Administration Medical
   Center, Saginaw, MI

PATIENT EDUCATION NEEDS
ASSESSMENT FOR PHYSICIANS

1. What input have you had regarding Patient Education at this
   Medical Center?   Name of Committees
      Committee Member_____
      Consult to a Committee_____   _____
      Informal discussions with staff_____   _____
      Discussions at physician meetings_____   _____

2. Do you write a specific order, on the physicians order sheet,
   for the patient to attend education class(es)?

      Yes_____
      No_____
      Sometimes_____

3. If you do not write a specific order for Patient Education, do
   you assume that other staff (e.g., nurses, dietitians, pharmacists,
   etc.) are referring patients to the appropriate classes?

      Yes_____
      No_____
      Haven't thought about it_____

4. What Patient Education programs are you aware of which are
   presently being offered for your patients?
   Please list:

5. Which of the following classes do you encourage your patients to
   attend?
      Diabetes_____   Alcohol_____
      Hypertension_____   Basic Nutrition_____
      COPD_____   No Added Salt_____
      Weight Reduction_____

6. Are there any Patient Education programs not presently available
   that you would like to see offered?

7. From feedback you have received from patients, in what ways have
   they benefited from the available Patient Education Programs?

8. In what ways are the patients prevented from benefiting from these programs?

9. Would it be helpful to you to have an orientation for the current Patient Education Programs and Activities available at this Medical Center?

        Yes_____
        No_____

10. If yes, would you prefer the orientation to be given:

        (a) at one of the monthly physician meetings_____

        (b) scheduled as an offering during Medical Grand Rounds_____

        (c) on an individual basis_____

11. Would you be interested in attending seminars regarding Patient Education if CME's in Category I are offered for physicians?

        Yes_____

        At this Medical Center_____

        Off Station_____

        No_____

12. Would you like to have more opportunity to participate in the Patient Education Programs? (Such as instructing, planning, or evaluating a program?)

        Yes_____

        No_____

        Possibly_____

13. Are there any suggestions you can offer to make these programs more beneficial for patients?

Scripps Memorial Hospital
LaJolla, CA

MEDICAL STAFF SURVEY

Physician Name:
Address: Phone:
Specialty: Target Population of Practice:
Board Certification:
Present University Affiliation: Teaching_____ Research_____
Are you accepting new patients?   Yes____ No____
What services do you offer:
        Insurance accepted?   Yes____ No____
            Private or Group   Yes____ No____   CHAMPUS   Yes____ No____
            Medi-Cal   Yes____ No____   MediCare   Yes____ No____

        Do you bill insurance companies directly?   Yes____ No____
Hours of Service: Routine_____   Emergency_____
Parking Facilities: Yes____ No____   Public Transportation Access: Yes____ No____

What are the major health problems you see in your practice?
    Major Problem   Age Group   % of Practice?
1.
2.
3.
4.
5.

In your opinion, what are the greatest health education needs of your patients?
1.
2.
3.
4.
5.

Do you have any organized patient education programs through your practice?
        Yes____ No____ If yes, please describe:

Do you refer patients to any health education programs in the community?
        Yes____ No____ If yes, which programs?

What community health education programs would you like to see implemented
at the health education center?

If you were to refer patients to the center for health education, what
information would you like to know prior to referral?

Would you like to be involved in educational programs at UTC Health Education
Center?   Yes____ No____
            Content development____ Delivery____ Advisor____ Panel Discussions____

How much time would you be willing to give to this activity?
    Hrs. per month   Hrs. per year

Reprinted with permission.

- 87 -

CASE STUDY 3

WORKING WITH PHYSICIANS THROUGH COMMITTEES

Change seldom occurs in a hospital without the involvement of at least one
committee. Cumbersome as this mechanism sometimes can be, it is often the
best way to communicate with and to gather input from individuals whose work
has relevance to a committee's purpose. This is no less true in the planning
and implementation of health promotion programs and in the involvement of
physicians in the process. To paraphrase an AHA manual on implementing
programs, an educator must identify and use mechanisms that ensure physician
involvement for several reasons. Such mechanisms--committees, task forces,
and ad hoc groups, for example--can help to gain support for health promotion
from other physicians, to establish priorities that coincide with physicians'
perception of need for programs, and to evaluate the benefit of such
programs.[1] No less important, physician committee members "can provide
valuable insights into how the hospital and their own departments work and can
identify effective ways to gain support not only for" health promotion in
general, but also for the program coordinator's role. "They can also introduce
the coordinator to professionals in their own departments and help legitimate
efforts of the coordinator to work with these staff."

Existing Health Promotion Committees

As Chapter 6 suggests, one logical point for physician involvement is a
hospital-wide committee that oversees one area of health promotion programming,
such as patient education. In addition to being one mechanism for physician
input into program planning, physician membership on such a broad-based
committee is often a good orientation to the organization and delivery of all
the services that are offered by a department. In turn, an awareness of these
matters can help physicians to better understand the need for coordination of
department activities and therefore to appreciate the role of the program
coordinator. Their support of the coordinator's role will often follow, as it
did at the Veterans Administration Medical Center in Saginaw, MI.

Before a patient education coordinator was appointed at the medical center,
recounts Margaret Bazeley, who assumed this position in early 1981, a
hospital-wide patient education committee consisting of chiefs of service
(department heads) was responsible for coordinating hospital-wide programming.
The development and delivery of programs was and continues to be largely
decentralized, with each relevant department responsible for its own programs.
A physician acted as consultant to the committee, but he did not always
participate in meetings nor was he a liaison to the rest of the medical staff.
A physician survey that Bazeley conducted (see Case Study 2, for further
details) revealed that the opportunities for enlisting physicians in patient
education programming that are available with a full-time, salaried medical
staff were not being used at the medical center. Physicians' responses
indicated a significant lack of awareness of all the patient education
services that were available or of the possibilities that existed for

developing other programs. Clearly, physicians needed to be better oriented to the patient education services before they could begin to support their use by patients. One of the first outcomes of the physician survey report was therefore the appointment of a physician as a full member of the hospital-wide patient education advisory committee. This action by the chief of the medical staff ensures that physician input is always available in patient education programming deliberations and that a physician will bring those issues to the attention of the rest of the medical staff.

Having only one point of formal contact with the medical staff--such as through a physician member of an advisory committee--may often be insufficient to the purpose of effective medical staff involvement in health promotion activities. For example, the medical staff may be too large for one physician to successfully act as liaison between the two groups. Or the medical staff may wish to assume more of an oversight function in the development of various population-specific programs. In these and other circumstances, educators seek out a variety of relationships with already existing medical staff committees. To find the best match between a particular committee's activities and the objectives of a given health promotion program, the following issues should be considered:[2]

- If the program is population-specific (e.g., cardiac rehabilitation), do the committee members represent those specialties whose patients will most likely benefit from the programs?

- Is the committee's influence in the institution such that it can significantly affect the development and delivery of the program?

- If the committee will be expected not only to review but also to develop some portions of program materials, does it have sufficient membership or a subcommittee mechanism to accomplish specific tasks for committee review?

- Do most committee members have a genuine commitment to working toward a consensus on program-related issues?

- Will the specific health promotion program objective that is added to its charges become a priority for committee members, or will previously established committee objectives take undue precedence?

- Does the committee's schedule coincide with the schedule that has been established for the health promotion program?

With these questions in mind, some obvious choices can be made when physician input is wanted for certain kinds of programs. For example, the development of a preoperative teaching program is a likely matter for review by the surgical committee. Sometimes a committee whose charges are clearly related to a program does not exist, but a clinical department can serve as a committee through its periodic meeetings. For example, the physician members of the obstetrics/gynecology department can act as a review panel for a childbirth education series. In a teaching institution, the possibilities for physician committee input into health promotion program efforts may be broader than those in a hospital that has only the traditional set of medical staff committees. Educators in teaching hospitals should therefore consider medical faculty committees as additional sources of input into program planning and development. Among them may be groups of physicians who are especially interested in newer forms of medical care delivery, such as preventive medicine, and may therefore be valuable advisors in health promotion programming.

The process of adding a charge to a medical staff committee's functions is very often formalized and defined in medical staff bylaws. Because the process differs somewhat from institution to institution, educators in search of an appropriate committee must not assume that their choice will necessarily coincide with that of the medical staff, or in particular, with that of the chief of staff, who often is the person who charges a committee with a particular set of objectives. It is wise, then, to get the advice of knowledgeable persons about the appropriateness of a relationship with various committees, to develop a list of preferences that can be supported in discussions with the chief of staff and administrators, and to be ready to accept the choice that is made on the department's behalf.

If no one medical staff committee seems entirely suited to the purpose of reviewing a particular issue, it may be that the issue requires multidisciplinary deliberation. For example, if an education department is given the task of developing a patient information booklet about the efficient use of an outpatient clinic's services, the project has relevance beyond physicians' relationships with their patients. Asking for a medical staff committee's formal approval of this kind of material is therefore not always necessary. It may be more appropriate to apply to a hospital-wide committee for its review of such materials; for example, a patient care committee or its equivalent normally has a broader scope than a medical staff committee but includes physicians in its membership.

Some hospital-wide committees have approval authority over the materials or programs that are submitted for their review, and a physician member who strongly opposes some change in health promotion programming may be able to sway other members' opinions and to block the change. If this happens consistently, it may be necessary to search out another route. At one institution, for example, a physician member of a medical records committee was consistently opposed to having patient education records included in medical charts in order to facilitate more efficient and standardized teaching. Repeated disapproval of the education department's attempts to have such forms incorporated into the medical record was serious enough to negate proposed improvements in the department's services to patients, and the matter was proposed instead to the medical care committee for resolution.

Forming New Committees

In the event there are no committees through which physicians can effectively be engaged in a hospital's health promotion activities, educators may find both the process of developing a committee and its result very valuable in increasing communication with a hospital's medical staff. Before this dialogue is begun, however, several issues should be reasonably well defined:

- What is the purpose of the committee (to advise in program planning, to review and comment about materials, to approve programs materials, to develop materials, or some combinations of these)?

- What is the proposed schedule for committee activities (periodic meetings, deadlines for committee action, terminations of committee activities, etc.)?

- How will the committee's work be organized and who will provide it with the necessary support (i.e., who will be responsible for calling meetings, for recording minutes, for preparing reports, etc.)?

- If it is a medical staff committee, to what degree will the health promotion staff be able to guide committee deliberations?

These and other such issues will most probably be subject to the approval of the chief of staff, if that physician is responsible for forming new committees of the medical staff and for assigning members of those committees. Members of the hospital's administrative staff and/or other physicians in medico-administrative positions may also be involved in the creation of new committees. Educators whose purpose in proposing a new committee of physicians is to seek their input and support must be ready to define what their needs are and to offer reasons for developing a committee structure that will support these needs. For example, an advisory committee is often a loosely structured body whose objective is deliberately defined in rather broad terms. It can help to assure a constant source of physician input into a department's overall or specific activities. From the physicians' viewpoint, their committee membership can be a reliable source of information about the hospital's activities in a certain area of interest. At United and Children's Hospital (St. Paul, MN), it was the administration's intent to develop a variety of occupational health and other health promotion services for businesses that would not simultaneously compete with the medical services that were being provided to them by physicians on the medical staff.[4] Barbara Johnson, director of health extension at the hospital, tried to reassure physicians in several ways--by visiting with them individually and explaining the hospital's plans for various services, by inviting them to add questions to the survey the hospital was planning to do among local manufacturing firms, and by asking them to join a loosely formed advisory group. Approximately 50 physicians who use the hospital are also associated in some degree as providers of medical care to the employees of local industry. Cool though most of them were to the hospital's beginning to offer some of these services to their industrial clients, many of the physicians did attend the periodic advisory group meetings.

It was during these early meetings that the physicians began to express some of the concerns they had about the services the hospital would be providing to their clients, Johnson reports. For example, they were worried that the quality of the services might not be high and that this would reflect negatively on themselves in the eyes of their industrial clients. Johnson responded to this anxiety by arranging for some of the providers of the various services to make presentations to the physician advisory group during some of its subsequent meetings. A respiratory therapist described the stop-smoking program and how it had succeeded in returning some workers to gainful employment. During another session, an occupational and a physical therapist described proposed work site evaluation for the purpose of diagnosing risk of injury to workers; the physicians were especially responsive to this proposal and tried to suggest ways to market the service to potential clients. This contrasted sharply with their previous position, which was to reject the idea of the hospital's approaching their clients without first consulting the physicians who provided them medical services.

Another barrier to the physicians' supporting the various health extension services the hospital offered was the fact that the hospital's fees for some support services (like pulmonary function testing) were often higher than other sources charged, so the physicians had no incentive to refer their clients' employees to the hospital. This issue was also discussed at advisory group meetings, and the physicians' input helped the hospital to restructure its fee schedule both to comply with third party reimbursement requirements and to offer support services to the physicians and their clients at a competitive cost. Positive outcomes of this kind have reaffirmed the value of the physician advisory group as a mechanism for dialogue and growing cooperation between the hospital and its medical staff.

When the situation calls for physicians' taking more responsibility than in the above example for steering the activities of a health promotion program, a more formally defined committee can be organized. At Paoli (PA) Memorial Hospital, the health education committee of the medical staff was formed some three years ago when the director of the health education department became aware that more physician input was needed in the development of the department's growing variety of programs. The request that such a committee be formed was made to the appropriate person on the hospital's administrative staff, who in turn made the proposal to the president of the medical staff; the proposal defined the objectives of the committee and explained the need for physician participation in program development. The president of the medical staff then appointed the committee members and the chairman and passed on the committee charges, according to the recommendations that were made by the director of health education. And a description of the committee was added to the medical staff bylaws. Some time later, the occupational health department also made a similar request for a medical staff committee to be formed to help develop the concept and the objectives of occupational health services at the hospital. Because the medical staff secretary was responsible for recording the minutes of the monthly meetings of both these committees, she noticed that their deliberations were beginning to focus on some common issues. The suggestion that the two committee interact to share their views on those issues was acceptable to both, especially because the committees had some overlapping membership. Currently, the committees routinely meet as one, with two physicians sharing the chairmanship; their membership includes 10 physicians, the director of the health education department, the coordinator of community education, and the vice president for general services.

The health education/occupational health committee has several purposes; it plans and evaluates programs and generally steers the activities of the two departments in directions that are acceptable to the medical staff. It does not, however, develop program content or materials. These tasks are accomplished by smaller, working committees or task forces.

For example, when the planning committee identified a series on nutrition as an objective for the following year, reports Julie A. Valenzano, R.N., coordinator of community education, the chairman of the health education committee suggested the names of physicians who would be willing and whose specialties would make them appropriate participants in developing and presenting the series to the community.[5] Six months before the series was to begin, the working committee--consisting of five physicians, three hospital dieticians, the coordinator of community education, and several dieticians from a local college--began to meet individually to identify and work on the segment of the series that each would be involved in presenting. For example, one session of the series was to discuss diet in coronary disease, and Valenzano met several times with a cardiologist and some of the dieticians to coordinate the development of that session.

No meetings were held that required all the committee members to attend, because the work was more efficiently accomplished with smaller group meetings. The brochure that advertised the series to the community listed all the committee members' names, giving each of them credit for the work they had done.

Some Guidelines for Working with Physician Committees

The experiences of the educators who report success in working with physicians on committees suggest that the general rules for effective committee functioning can also be applied here:

- Be prepared. The first meeting of the committee is especially important, for it may set the long-term tone of the group and help to shape much of its activities. If a physician is to be the chairperson of the committee, help that individual to develop an agenda, background materials, and any other information that will permit the first meeting to run smoothly. If the physicians on the committee are not very familiar with the general issues that are relevant to the committee's objectives, introduce some of this information at each meetings, but also define some area to which they can apply their own special knowledge and skill.

- Out of respect for the limited time all committee members have to offer, be brief and encourage others to be brief, when this is appropriate.

- Don't schedule more meetings than are necessary. Make certain meetings begin and end on time.

. Anticipate the requirements of program development deadlines and try to match them as closely as possible with the normal meeting schedules of the committees that may need to be involved in program development and/or review.

These guidelines seem to be simple enough, yet they are essential in effectively coordinating work by committee. The form of the committee has come to be maligned not so much because the form itself tends to confound a groups' ability to accomplish its purpose, but because the group sometimes lets the meeting become its purpose. No matter how widespread this kind of inefficient use of committee time may be even among a hospital's medical staff committees, educators should try to avoid it in their dealings with physician committees in particular. Besides being a refreshing change, this approach may offer additional evidence to physicians that their participation is indeed an essential part of a valuable and productive relationship.

References

1. American Hospital Association. Implementing Patient Education in the Hospital. Chicago: the AHA, 1979.

2. Bazeley, M. Personal communication, June 28, 1983.

3. Implementing Patient Education.

4. Johnson, B. Personal communication, June 27, 1983.

5. Valenzano, J. Personal communication, June 30, 1983.

APPENDIXES

ORGANIZATIONAL CONTACTS FOR PROGRAM EXAMPLES CITED IN TEXT

APPLETON MEMORIAL HOSPITAL
1818 North Meade Street
Appleton, WI 54911

Susan Lebergen
Community Relations Representative

BAPTIST HOSPITAL OF MIAMI, INC.
8900 North Kendall Drive
Miami, FL 33176

Leah S. Kinnaird, R.N., M.S.
Director of Patient and
    Community Education

BAPTIST MEMORIAL HOSPITAL
899 Madison Avenue
Memphis, TN 38146

Joy Lomax Martin
Patient Education Coordinator

BRACKENRIDGE HOSPITAL
601 E. 15 Street
Austin, TX 78701

Carolyn Hinckley Boyle
Community Wellness Director
Department of Community Relations

BRYAN MEMORIAL HOSPITAL
4848 Sumner Street
Lincoln, NE 68506

Loretta Olson, R.N.
Patient Teaching Coordinator

CENTER FOR HEALTH EDUCATION, INC.
Coggins Building
1204 Maryland Avenue
Baltimore, MD 21201

Carmine M. Valente, Ph.D.
Executive Director

COLUMBUS CHILDREN'S HOSPITAL
700 Children's Drive
Columbus, OH 43205

Rose Marie McCormick
Director, Homegoing Education and
    Literature Program

DAY KIMBALL HOSPITAL
320 Pomfret Street
Putnam, CT 06260

Dena Baskin, R.N.
Coordinator, Patient Education

DECATUR MEMORIAL HOSPITAL
2300 N. Edward Street
Decatur, IL 62526

Diane Jensen
Assistant Director of Nursing

DUKE UNIVERSITY MEDICAL CENTER
EMPLOYEE OCCUPATIONAL HEALTH SERVICE
Box 2914
Durham, NC 27710

George Jackson, M.D.
Director

EAST TENNESSEE CHILDREN'S HOSPITAL
2018 Clinch Avenue
Knoxville, TN 37916

Laura Borden, R.N.
Child Life Coordinator

EASTON HOSPITAL
CARL AND EMILY WELLER CENTER
   FOR HEALTH EDUCATION
2009 Lehigh Street
Easton, PA 18042

James A. Hruban
Executive Director

EL CAMINO HOSPITAL
2500 Grant Road
Mountain View, CA 94042

Mary Woodrow
Director, Health Management Services

GENERAL VENTURA COUNTY HOSPITAL
3291 Loma Vista Road
Ventura, CA 93009

Robert M. Huff, M.P.H.
Director of Patient Education

GRADY MEMORIAL HOSPITAL
80 Butler Street, S.E.
Atlanta, GA 30335

Kathleen Dobberstein
Patient Education Coordinator

GROUP HEALTH COOPERATIVE (GHC)
   OF PUGET SOUND
200 Fifteenth Avenue, East
Seattle, WA 98112

George A. Orr III
Director, Center for Health Promotion

HASCO
P.O. Box 343800
Coral Gables, FL 33114

Patricia Blanco, R.N., M.P.H.
Risk Management Consultant

HITCHCOCK CLINIC
Hanover, NH 03755

Joann Kairys
Health Education Program Coordinator

INGHAM MEDICAL CENTER
401 W. Greenlawn Avenue
Lansing, MI 48909

Sue A. Stock
Chief of Occupational Therapy

JACKSON CLINIC
30 S. Henry
Madison, WI 53703

Pat Herje
Director of Health Education

KAISER-PERMANENTE MEDICAL CENTER
280 W. MacArthur Boulevard
Oakland, CA 92103

Pamela Jean Larson
Director of Health Education

KETTERING MEDICAL CENTER
3535 Southern Boulevard
Kettering, OH 45429

David J. Kinsey, M.A.
Director, Media Department

MADISON GENERAL HOSPITAL
202 S. Park Street
Madison, WI   53715

John Mullin
Director of Exercise Physiology Services

MERCY MEDICAL CENTER
16th Avenue at Milwaukee Street
Denver, CO   80206

Donald Iverson, Ph.D.
Director of Health Promotion/
   Disease Prevention (HP/DP)

MONTEFIORE HOSPITAL AND MEDICAL CENTER
111 E. 210th Street
Bronx, NY   10467

Josephine Laventhol
Director of Patient Education

MOUNT AUBURN HOSPITAL
330 Mount Auburn Street
Cambridge, MA   02238

Dorie Hauss, R.N.
Cardiac Rehabilitation Clinical Specialist

NORTH CENTRAL REGIONAL MEDICAL
   EDUCATION CENTER
VETERANS ADMINISTRATION
5445 Minnehaha Avenue South
Minneapolis, MN   55417

Anne Stechmann, M.A.
Coordinator, Patient Health Education

PAOLI MEMORIAL HOSPITAL
Lancaster Pike
Paoli, PA   19301

Julie A. Valenzano, RN
Coordinator of Community Education
215/648-1000

PRESBYTERIAN-ST. LUKE'S MEDICAL CENTER
1850 Williams Street
Denver, CO   80218

Michael D. Chisholm
Director, Community Programs

ST. ELIZABETH HOSPITAL MEDICAL CENTER
1044 Belmont Avenue
Youngstown, OH   44501

Sr. Mary Carl Kotheimer
Director, Nursing Service

ST. JOHN'S HOSPITAL
P.O. Box 1688
Salina, KS   67401

Peg Romine
Patient Education Coordinator

ST. JOSEPH HOSPITAL
601 North 30th Street
Omaha, NE   68131

Joseph J. Fanucchi, M.D.
Director, Occupational Health Service

ST. JOSEPH MERCY HOSPITAL
Route #3
Centerville, IA   52544

Kathy Powers, R.N.
Patient Education Coordinator

ST. LOUIS PARK MEDICAL CENTER
5000 West Thirty-Ninth Street
Minneapolis, MN   55416

Paul B. Batalden, M.D.
Program Director
Health Services Research Center

ST. MARY'S HOSPITAL
1800 E. Lake Shore Drive
Decatur, IL 62525

Judy O'Connor
Instructor, Nursing Staff Development
  Office

ST. MARY-ROGERS MEMORIAL HOSPITAL
12th and West Walnut Street
Rogers, AR 72756

Connie Elzey
Administrative Assistant

ST. VINCENT HOSPITAL AND
  HEALTH CARE CENTER
ST. VINCENT WELLNESS CENTERS
2001 W. 86th Street
Indianapolis, IN 46260

Barbara Burke
Assistant Manager

ST. VINCENT'S HOSPITAL AND
  MEDICAL CENTER
9205 S.W. Barnes Road
Portland, OR 97225

Barbara Main
Director of Educational Services

SCRIPPS MEMORIAL HOSPITAL
P.O. Box 28
LaJolla, CA 92038

Christine Brown
Program Director, The Well Being

SISTERS OF ST. MARY FAMILY
  MEDICINE CENTER
2900 Baltimore
Kansas City, MO 64108

John Renner, M.D.
Director

STORMONT-VAIL REGIONAL
  MEDICAL CENTER
1500 Southwest 10th Street
Topeka, KS 66606

Ted Warren, Ph.D.
Director, Division of Education

UNITED AND CHILDREN'S HOSPITALS
333 N. Smith Street
Minneapolis, MN 55102

Barbara Johnson
Health Education Director

UNITED GENERAL HOSPITAL
P.O. Box 410
Sedro Woolley, WA 98284

M. Daniel Sloan
Health Promotion Coordinator

UNIVERSITY OF CALIFORNIA, LOS ANGELES
School of Medicine
Center for the Health Sciences
Los Angeles, CA 90024

Charles E. Lewis, M.D.
Professor of Medicine

UNIVERSITY OF MARYLAND HOSPITAL
Redwood and Greene Streets
Baltimore, MD 21201

Linda Hines, R.N., M.S.
Clinical Specialist, Ambulatory Nursing

UNIVERSITY OF TEXAS CANCER CENTER
M. D. ANDERSON HOSPITAL AND TUMOR
  INSTITUTE
6723 Bertner
Houston, TX 77030

Katherine Crosson, M.P.H.
Director, Patient Education Section

VETERANS ADMINISTRATION MEDICAL CENTER
1500 Weiss Street
Saginaw, MI 48602

Margaret A. Bazeley
Patient Health Education Coordinator

WESLEY MEDICAL CENTER
550 N. Hillside
Wichita, KS 67214

D. Cramer Reed, M.D.
President, HEALTH STRATEGIES, INC.

Appendix B

PROJECTS ON INCREASING PHYSICIAN INVOLVEMENT
IN HEALTH PROMOTION

The following projects have been included in this document because they are specifically designed to help physicians assume more responsibility in health promotion; some of these projects are also intended to develop materials that will help physicians to incorporate health promotion into their patient care practices. The list is by no means all inclusive, but it does represent several substantial efforts, the results of which promise to be applicable in a wide variety of settings.

Center for Educational Development in Health
Boston University School of Medicine
80 E. Concord Street
Boston, MA 02118

Hannelore Vanderschmidt, Ph.D.
Director, Curriculum Development Project
617/353-4528

Originally intended to develop a syllabus to teach preventive medicine to undergraduate medical students, the project has modified materials so that they can be used in continuing medical education for various primary care practitioners. Materials are divided into three modules: one on the epidemiologic basis for prevention, another on the management of a preventive medical practice, and a third on clinical application of the principles of health maintenance. These materials as well as the consulting services of the center's staff are available to those who are interested in providing continuing medical education programs on these topics.

Center for Health Education, Inc.
1204 Maryland Avenue
Baltimore, MD 21201

Carmine M. Valente, Ph.D.
Executive Director
301/837-2705

This organization is a private, non-profit corporation established in 1982 as a joint venture of the Medical and Chirurgical Faculty of the State of Maryland and Blue Cross and Blue Shield of Maryland. The purpose of the center is to encourage and assist the physician and organized medicine to take an increased leadership role in health education and health promotion activities in Maryland. One way of accomplishing this purpose is through the development of continuing education programs for physicians "in the techniques of promoting healthy lifestyles among their patients." An example of a recent program is a two-session course taught by physicians to help increase adherence rates among hypertensives by increasing physician skills in communication and hypertension education and management.

The Health Promotion/Disease Prevention Program
Mercy Medical Center
16th Avenue at Milwaukee Street
Denver, CO 80206

Donald Iverson, Ph.D.
Program Director
303/393-3096

This program is located within the hospital's family medicine residency
program; one of its objectives, therefore, is to develop a health promotion/
disease prevention curriculum to be used to teach family medicine residents.
The program plans to develop 24 modules to use in the program and later to
disseminate in compilation as protocols that physicians can use in their
practice. Five of the modules are applicable to a variety of health problems;
they cover medical compliance, use of non-physician medical alternatives,
principles of persuasive communication, and principles of patient learning/
behavior change. The fifth module offers specific guidelines for integrating
health promotion/disease prevention into physicians' practice settings. The
other 19 modules cover such topics as accident prevention, alcohol and drug
use, chronic pain management, human sexuality, self-care, parenting,
immunization, and others. Plans to publish these modules for wider
distribution in the field are being made as this book goes to press.

Health Promotion Research Project
Department of Family Medicine
Wayne State University
Gordon H. Scott Hall of Basic
  Medical Sciences
540 E. Canfield Avenue
Detroit, MI 48201

Joseph Hess, M.D.
Principal Investigator

Ann Gorton, Ph.D.
Project Administrator
312/577-1406

A four-year study funded by the W. K. Kellogg Foundation, this project is
designed to evaluate the cost effectiveness of two methods to reduce risk
from smoking, hypertension, dyslipidemia, sedentary lifestyle, and obesity.
The effectiveness of appropriate patient education by a health educator will
be compared with the effectiveness of patients' discussing risk reduction with
their own health care provider. Persons interested in the results of this
project may ask to be included in a mailing list for the final report, which
will probably include recommendations to physicians on the interventions they
can use in their office practices.

Health-Styles
Family Practice Research Project
Memorial Hospital
7777 Southwest Freeway, Suite 933
Houston, TX 77074

John Sims
Project Director
713/776-5305

Funded by the W. K. Kellogg Foundation, this project is designed to evaluate
the effectiveness of materials and methods for teaching physicians and helping
physicians to incorporate health promotion principles into their practice
settings. The project has just begun its first evaluation stage, which will
last 18 months and will study the effectiveness of interventions related to
four risk factors in cardiovascular disease: obesity, lack of exerise,
smoking, and stress. The Family Practice Center, in which family practice
residents are trained, will be the site for the project. Although the
materials that the project has and will continue to develop will not be
available until all phases of evaluation are completed, periodic progress
reports may be obtained by those who are interested in learning about the
project's positive and negative experiences in teaching physicians to use
various interventions.

INSURE
Lifestyle Preventive Health Services Project (LPHS)
330 Park Avenue, South
New York, NY 10010

Donald N. Logsdon, M.D.
Director
212/578-8176

The intent of this three-year feasibility study begun in 1980 was to define
age-specific procedures and packages of preventive health services, including
patient education; to develop related protocols and educational interventions
and to implement these with the help of primary care physicians at group
practice study sites; and to study the short-term effects of the project on
physicians and patients. The impact of preventive services on third party
payors as well as the costs of these services will also be studied. The
project developed a variety of materials, including a comprehensive manual,
which project staff used to teach participating physicians LPHS guidelines,
directions for using patient encounter forms, and strategies for patient
communication and education. As the feasibility project draws to a close,
interested health professionals may obtain from INSURE staff descriptions of
the study and of the contents of the manual as well as an outline of LPHS
guidelines. Plans for future distribution of the manual itself await
completion of the project, although it is anticipated that a continuing
medical education program may eventually be developed on the basis of this
study.

Projects in Health Promotion
American Medical Association
535 North Dearborn Street
Chicago, IL 60610

William Carlyon, Ph.D.
Director, Health Education Program
312/751-6588

As this book goes to press, the American Medical Association (AMA) is working on several projects that are related to physician involvement in health promotion. One of these is intended to produce a publication on guidelines for physicians' incorporating patient education into their practices in various ambulatory care settings. This publication will be used in conjunction with a continuing series of AMA education programs for physicians on marketing their practices to their communities. The AMA is also planning a survey of state and local medical societies to assess their involvement in various health promotion activities; a report of survey findings will probably be available by early 1984. The staff of the department of health education is also available on a continuing basis to help physicians identify appropriate resources for patient education and health promotion and to provide copies of some of the resources that are in printed form.

APPENDIX C

HEALTH PROMOTION REFERENCES FOR PHYSICIANS

1. American Academy of Family Physicians. DUET--Drug Use Education Tips.
    Kansas City, MO.

    Based on materials developed by the United States Pharmacopeia (USP),
    this patient education program provides physicians information about
    drugs that can be readily passed on to and understood by patients.

2. American Medical Association. Patient Medication Instructions. Chicago,
    IL.

    Called PMIs, these instruction sheets are meant to be given to patients
    at the time of prescribing; the information they contain is based on AMA
    Drug Evaluations and on information from the USP.

3. Batalden, P. B., O'Connor, J. P. Quality Assurance in Ambulatory Care.
    Germantown, MD: Aspen Systems Corporation, 1980.

    Specific guidelines and worksheets for implementing quality assurance in
    ambulatory care settings.

4. "But, Doctor, You Said..." Viewer's Guide. Metropolitan Life Insurance
    Company, New York, NY. 1978.

    A film and discussion guide for teaching communication skills to
    physicians, nurses, and other health professionals.

5. Carlyon, P. Physician's Guide to the School Health Curriculum Process.
    Third Edition. Chicago, IL: American Medical Association, 1983.

    A basic orientation to a philosophy of health instruction, as well as
    detailed guidelines for incorporating health education into school
    curricula.

6. Griffith, H. W. Drug Information for Patients. Philadelphia, PA: W. B.
    Saunders Co., 1978.

    A collection of drug information and instruction sheets that can be
    removed from the loose-leaf binder, photocopied, and given to patients
    to supplement one-to-one instruction.

7. Griffith, H. W. and others. <u>Information and Instructions for Pediatric Patients</u>. Tucson, AZ: Winter Publishing Company, 1980.

   Loose-leaf bound information sheets designed to be copied and given to pediatric patients and their parents; addresses more than 250 common pediatric problems.

8. <u>Instructional Modules to Teach Primary Care Residents to Educate Patients</u>. D.H.H.S. Contract No. 232-79-0026. Project Director, Marion Field Fass, Sc.D., University of Wisconsin. Department of Family Medicine and Practice, Madison, WI. 1981.

   Six modules designed to teach communication and teaching skills, psychosocial aspects of patient education, the planning and implementing of short-term patient education strategies, principles of health promotion and behavior change, and the incorporation of patient education into practice.

9. Morgan, P. <u>Nutrition in Family Medicine: A Resource Guide for the Clinical Setting</u>. Sponsored by the University of California, San Francisco, Area Health Education Centers (AHEC), a project of the University supported in part by DHEW Contract HRA-232-79-0006. 1979.

   A manual to aid primary care practitioners to screen for nutritional problems, assess patients' nutritional status, and to identify resources for nutrition counseling and information.

10. <u>Patient Education: A Handbook for Teachers</u>. Report of the National Task Force on Training Family Physicians in Patient Education. Printed by The Society of Teachers of Family Medicine, 1740 West 92nd Street, Kansas City, MO 64114. December 1979.

    A document intented for use in teaching the principles of patient education to family practice residents. It discusses the deveopment of patient teaching skills, offers guidelines for incorporating patient education into office practice, and includes references to many useful resources.

11. <u>Patient Education in Practice</u>. An ASIM Guide for Physicians and their staff. Order from the American Society of Internal Medicine, 2550 M Street, N.W., Suite 620, Washington, DC 20037. August 1981.

    A brief guide for practicing physicians and their office staff on patient education techniques and educational resources.

12. <u>Patient Education Primer</u>. A Guide for Practicing Physicians. Order from The Society of Teachers of Family Medicine, 1740 West 92nd Street, Kansas City, MO 64114.

    An excerpt from <u>Patient Education: A Handbook for Teachers</u>, prepared specifically for practicing family physicians interested in increasing the emphasis that they place on patient education in their practice.

13. Patient Education in the Primary Care Setting. Proceedings of the Fifth
    Annual Conference. Kansas City, MO. September 20-21, 1982. (For
    information availability of this proceedings contact Sisters of St. Mary
    Regional Family Practice Residency, Kansas City, MO.)

    The conference proceedings include discussions on counselling patients
    about their medications, on using electronic media in patient education,
    and various other issues.

14. The Physician's Guide: How to Help Your Hypertensive Patients Stop
    Smoking. U.S. Department of Health and Human Services, Public Health
    Service, National Institutes of Health, Bethesda, MD, 1983.

    Guidelines for easily incorporating minimal as well as expanded smoking
    cessation procedures into the care of hypertensive patients.

15. Physician's Guide to Patient Education Materials. Pennsylvania Medical
    Society, 20 Erford Road, Lemoyne, PA 17043. 1982.

    A brief set of guidelines for evaluating and choosing the most appropriate
    materials and programs for teaching patients; also provides a list of
    selected sources of materials.

16. Taylor, R. B., and others. Health Promotion: Principles and Clinical
    Applications. Norwalk, CT: Appleton-Century-Crofts, 1982.

    A multi-authored text that is intended to help primary care providers to
    understand the principles of health promotion, determine the health
    promotion needs of individuals and their families, prescribe appropriate
    health promoting interventions, and maintain continuing supervision in
    accord with up-to-date scientific data.